DE-STRESSING DOCTORS

A self-management guide

Valerie Sutherland
Chartered Occupational Psychologist, Surrey

Cary L Cooper
University of Manchester Institute of Science
and Technology

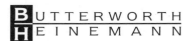
BUTTERWORTH
HEINEMANN

EDINBURGH LONDON NEW YORK OXFORD
PHILADELPHIA ST LOIUS SYDNEY TORONTO 2003

BUTTERWORTH-HEINEMANN
An imprint of Elsevier Science Limited

First published 2003

ISBN 0 7506 8783 5

British Library Cataloguing in Publication Data
A catalogue record for this book is available from the British Library

Library of Congress Cataloging in Publication Data
A catalog record for this book is available from the Library of Congress

Note
Medical knowledge is constantly changing. Standard safety precautions must be followed, but as new research and clinical experience broaden our knowledge, changes in treatment and drug therapy may become necessary or appropriate. Readers are advised to check the most current product information provided by the manufacturer of each drug to be administered to verify the recommended dose, the method and duration of administration, and contraindications. It is the responsibility of the practitioner, relying on experience and knowledge of the patient, to determine dosages and the best treatment for each individual patient. Neither the Publisher nor the authors assumes any liability for any injury and/or damage to persons or property arising from this publication.

The Publisher

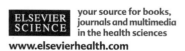

ELSEVIER
SCIENCE
your source for books,
journals and multimedia
in the health sciences
www.elsevierhealth.com

The
publisher's
policy is to use
paper manufactured
from sustainable forests

Printed in China

DE-STRESSING
DOCTORS

A self-management guide

For Butterworth Heinemann:

Publishing Manager: Heidi Allen
Development Editor: Robert Edwards
Project Manager: Morven Dean
Design: George Ajayi
Illustration Manager: Bruce Hogarth

Contents

Preface

This self-management guide aims to help doctors deal effectively with the strains and pressures that are an inevitable part of working as a professional in medical practice - we have described this as 'de-stressing doctors'. We use the term doctor to refer to any person who is licensed to practice medicine and working in general practice, as a family doctor, or in either a hospital or clinic healthcare environment, as a generalist, specialist or consultant practitioner. However, it is also acknowledged that the role of the doctor extends beyond the practice of medicine per se. Typically, the contemporary role of the medical practitioner embraces a wide range of social, business and management skills and abilities. From research evidence and discussions with doctors it is evident that many perceive this feature of professional life to be mainly responsible for creating strain and pressure, rather than the actual practice of medicine itself. Therefore, there is a strong need to include such elements in a comprehensive stress management, self-help guide for doctors because medicine is a science **and** a business.

The individual who chooses to become a doctor is probably the sort of person who seeks a challenging and demanding job. As patients we bring our health problems to our doctor and expect the highest standards of care and treatment. Both parties in this relationship want a successful outcome. It means that the doctor, as a carer of other people, is required to maintain a constant high level of performance. Consequently the nature of the job exposes the doctor to potential pressure. While pressure can be positive and motivational, under certain conditions this pressure can become negative. The term 'stress' is used to describe this state-stress is unwanted pressure. It is important to clarify what we mean by stress because it has become a contentious issue. The meaning is not always clear and some have suggested that stress does not exist because you cannot see it or measure it. Our view on this is simple. We use the word 'stress' as a way of discussing all the events, conditions and situations that exist in the life of the medical practitioner to create a situation whereby, for one of many reasons, the doctor is unable to perform to the best of his or her ability.

In many ways, doctors face pressures similar to other professionals because the contemporary work environment is characterised by constant change. Over the last five decades of the twentieth century the nature of society and medical practice work has altered dramatically, thereby creating stress conditions for both doctor and patient. Strategic and radical change in attitudes to health care, health care arrangements and services has affected the nature of the doctor–patient relationship. Doctors often feel that they no longer have the high levels of autonomy or control previously enjoyed by the profession, and consequently job satisfaction and moral levels have been eroded. Employer demands and financial constraints typically create shortages in material and staff resources. This forces restrictions on medical practice and can create conflict and negative emotions for the doctor. While the doctor does the best for a patient, it is often within certain unwanted limitations. Constant exposure to this type of work situation, generically described as 'stress' or unwanted pressure, has been linked to a variety of adverse physical, emotional or behavioural conditions, which in the long term can have a negative affect on job performance, work satisfaction and quality of life of the doctor. Since it is acknowledged that exposure to mismanaged stress can, under certain conditions, also have a negative impact on physical and psychological health, it is crucial that doctors are able to effectively manage the stress that is inherent in the job. Thus, the word stress is used to describe these negative work and living conditions, and stress management techniques are used to explore ways of avoiding or mitigating a potentially stressful and damaging situation.

Eliminating the source stress, or stress agent, is acknowledged as the most effective approach to stress management. However, this is not always a realistic option in dealing with many of the sources of stress intrinsic to the job of the medical practitioner and their support staff. Therefore, we contend that it is necessary to manage stress and learn how to cope with it in an effective manner to avoid becoming a casualty or victim of mismanaged stress. In simple terms, stress management works by creating optimal conditions and through improved self-awareness. The benefits of successful stress management are both economic and humanistic, including professional satisfaction and high job performance. Through the mechanism of stress management the doctor is able to enjoy a better quality of life, health and happiness and satisfaction as a professional in medical practice. It is about gaining and maintaining work-life balance.

In the following chapters we offer guidance and advice for the self-management of stress among doctors and offer the 'Triple A' approach as a strategy that can be used by the individual, a group or team of doctors, or a healthcare environment such as a group practice, clinic or hospital department. 'Triple A' stands for:

AWARENESS
ANALYSIS
ACTION

Therefore, in Part 1, 'The face of stress' we raise AWARENESS by providing a definition of what we mean by the word 'stress', and why and how it is damaging in its consequences in medical practice. A transactional model of stress is described and provided to guide the process of stress diagnosis or ANALYSIS among doctors and their staff and colleagues. This forms the topic of Chapter 2 and includes practical ways of identifying stress and examples of diagnostic studies into the nature of stress amongst medical practitioners. Only when we recognise and understand a stress problem can we take the necessary and appropriate action for the management of stress. Therefore, the remainder of this self-management guide is devoted to ACTION and options for the management of stress in medical practice, because there is not one problem, neither is there one solution.

In Part 2, Chapter 3 addresses the issue of time management for doctors, while Chapter four provides practical suggestions for creating a more effective and stress-free medical practice environment for doctors and their staff. Since we acknowledge that stress is not just out there in the environment, and must be perceived to be a source of stress, Part 3 considers the relationship between behaviour and stress. It explains how and why certain patterns of behaviour can create or exacerbate a stress problem. Therefore, Chapter five specifically addresses the topic of aggression and stress, while Chapter six examines another stress prone personality, namely the Type A coronary prone pattern of behaviour. Both chapters offer guidance on the recognition, measurement and management of these potentially damaging styles of behaviour among doctors. Specific stress management strategies include: anger and conflict management; this incorporates the issue of assertiveness as a stress control strategy; dealing with criticism; role negotiation; and key points in the control of Type A behaviour.

In Part 4, Chapter 7, a personal action plan is provided with guidance on successful steps to stress control. Finally, in Chapter 8 we offer of a range of strategies to help the individual doctor respond to stress in a positive manner. These include: relaxation techniques and breathing exercises; venting steam; cognitive methods in the management of stress – that is, dealing with faulty thinking; the role of social support in stress management; exercise and stress control; career breaks – that is 'getting off the hot seat'

Since the work demands of the medical practitioner include management and administrative demands, this aspect of the medical practitioner job role is addressed. In addition, we acknowledge that doctors do not work in a social vacuum and so this guide refers to the interaction and relationships between doctors, their colleagues, medical support staff and the many non-medical personnel who interact with medical practitioners on a regular basis. Thus, the aim of this book is to help doctors to become their own stress manager and to produce a simple action plan for the management of stress.

part ONE

The face of stress

It has been said that stress is like 'love' and 'electricity' – we all have experiences of these things but somehow find it difficult to explain such phenomena because they cannot be seen or held in our hands. Indeed, if asked, a group of doctors would probably each describe these concepts of stress, love and electricity in very different ways. Therefore, the purpose of the next two chapters is to raise awareness about the nature of this thing called 'stress', and to explain how and why it is damaging in its consequences. It is important to know what it is AND what it is not, because of the misunderstandings that seem to exist! This is a vital part of the process of stress management. Whilst we tend to use the word 'stress' in a generic way, it will be seen that stress is a multi-faceted concept. There is neither one problem nor one solution. Identifying the best option available for the management of stress is contingent upon a clear understanding of what we mean by 'stress'. This is the topic of Chapter one. Effective stress management is also dependent upon the ability to accurately diagnose and assess our stress-related problems. The stress audit process and the nature of stress among hospital and general practice doctors are discussed in Chapter two.

Stress is not a four-letter word

To successfully manage stress we must define what we mean by the term 'stress', identify it and understand the effects of exposure to it. It is also necessary to recognize how and why stress is damaging in its consequences. To help and guide this AWARENESS-raising process, a transactional model of stress is used to explain why exposure to certain conditions and situations can have an adverse impact on the performance, health and quality of life of the doctor.

Stress – whipping boy or reality?

The word 'stress' is part of our everyday language. A patient will readily use the word 'stress' to discuss a problem with a doctor. The doctor understands the word stress as a biological, neurological or hormonal response, ·and recognizes the emotional implications associated with the phenomena. However, we tend to use the word interchangeably and in distinctly different ways, thereby creating confusion in the process of stress management. For example, the word 'stress' is used to refer to:

- a perceived state or condition. For example, we say, 'I am feeling really stressed today'
- a symptom that we experience. This can refer to a wide variety of physical or emotional feelings, or our behavioural reaction when stressed, such as, feeling depressed,

anxious, having insomnia, a headache, or muscle tension etc.

- the perceived cause of our condition or symptom. For example, an emergency has caused the evening surgery to be disrupted, resulting in the need to work even later than usual.

As we have already said, there are problems about a common definition of the word 'stress', if indeed one exists. We also question whether the word itself is useful. Terms such as, 'stress', 'pressure' and 'strain' are all used to describe feelings, emotions or situations. The layperson seems quite able to identify with the concept of stress and has an appetite to know more. It is a need that is served eagerly by the press and media. Without a doubt, certain individuals hope to use the litigation process to make a quick profit by citing work stress. This can create problems for us in the effective management of stress because it is wrongly blamed for every ill and seen as the cause of all work-related problems. It has become a 'whipping boy' and is certainly misunderstood. Indeed, some have described stress as 'the back-pain of the 21st century', and it is common for us to view stress only in negative terms, or to deny that any stress problem exists. It is also synonymous with an inability to cope, particularly in macho industries and workplaces. By necessity, doctors hide their stress from patients and, in our experience, usually from each other. The prevalence of such views and attitudes are detrimental to the effective management of stress in the work environment. It leads to the creation of a negative work culture wherein people hide problems and their ill health until they become victims and casualties of exposure to stress. It is neither useful nor cost-effective to simply put the blame for not coping on the individual doctor or their staff and assistants. Neither should we continue to put the onus for change on the individual in healthcare work. Effective stress management requires us to examine the work environment and identify the barriers to effective job performance, satisfaction and well-being. There is a need to discourage a negative view of stress and to provide encouragement for active and positive management of the strains and pressures that are an inevitable part of the medical practice today. The stress process is dynamic, not a static situation or condition, and so it is realistic to acknowledge that all doctors are more or less vulnerable to stress at certain times in their lives. The ability to recognize this and know how to deal with it is a key stress-management skill.

Not all stress is bad!

It is not the intention or purpose of this book to provide a detailed account of the biological, neurological or hormonal nature of stress. Such an account written by psychologists is unlikely to satisfy or inform a medical practitioner. However, it is necessary to set down our premise and certain key points in order to provide a framework to guide the stress-management process.

First, it is vital that we acknowledge that NOT ALL STRESS IS BAD. Hans Selye, the 'father' of stress research, said that the only person without stress was a dead person! By this Selye (1976) meant that stress is an inevitable part of being alive, and should be viewed as, 'stimulation to growth and development . . . it is challenge and variety, it is the spice of life'. Figure 1 illustrates this concept and the view that stress is essential for optimal performance. We need a certain degree of stress in order to perform, but accept it in excess and it can cause job burnout. The condition that we describe as 'rust-out' can also occur when medical practitioners feel that their skills and abilities are not being utilized to their satisfaction, or the work environment is perceived as boring. Apathy and loss of morale are both symptoms of job underload or rust-out.

Hans Selye used the word 'stress' to describe arousal of the central nervous system. So, stress can be defined as *any* stimulus, event or demand impacting on the sensory nervous system. When an imbalance exists between a perceived demand (that is, the stimulus) and our perceived

Medical Practitioners–Stress and Performance
Not all Stress is Bad!

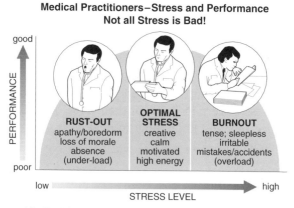

Figure 1.1   Medical Practitioners – stress and performance: not all stress is bad!

ability to meet that demand, we will experience a state of stress. Stress, therefore, as Figure 1 shows, can be both underload and overload, and is described as 'unwanted pressure'. It becomes manifest when we feel that a situation is out of our control or when we feel unable to cope with the demand placed upon us.

The damaging nature of the stress response

The response to stress has been described as the 'fight or flight syndrome' (Cannon 1935). It prepares our body to take action by increasing sympathetic activity via the secretion of catecholamines. Internal physiological changes initiated by the hormones, adrenaline (US name: epinephrine), noradrenaline (US name: norepinephrine) and cortisol, provide us with energy from the metabolism of fat and glucose. This causes an increased supply of oxygen (another energy source) to muscles through the rise in the number of red blood cells in the circulation, increased blood flow to the muscles, with reduced blood flow to the skin and the gut. Table 1.1 illustrates the physiological changes that occur in response to a stressor stimulus.

At such times we will experience the effects of the physiological response to arousal, such as, a dry mouth; 'butterflies' in the stomach, indigestion or nausea as non-essential

Table 1.1 Actions of adrenaline, noradrenaline and cortisol

Actions of adrenaline (USA – epinephrine) and noradrenaline (USA – norepinephrine)
- Fat and glucose mobilized from store – glucose stored as glycogen in the liver is released to provide energy for muscular and brain action
- Spleen contracts – circulate more red blood cells
- Blood clots more easily – blood supplies are redirected from the skin and viscera to provide an improved supply to the brain and skeletal muscles – gut activity slows
- Goose pimples – hair stands erect
- Arms, legs and body-wall muscles tense
- Heart beats faster – blood pressure increases
- Brain alert – quick decisions
- Pupils dilate
- Hearing more acute
- Breathing rapid/deeper
- Kidneys – reduced urine formation
- Saliva reduces

Actions of cortisol
- Sensitizes organs to adrenaline, and noradrenaline
- NORMAL levels enhance immune activity – supply of blood lymphocytes is increased to combat the impact of injury and infection from wounds
- Mobilizes glucose and fats from store
- Reduces inflammation
- Aids wound healing
- Reduces allergic reactions
- But, EXCESSIVE levels suppress the immune system

digestive processes slow down or cease; muscle tension caused by catecholamines, this muscle tension is needed to keep muscles partially contracted ready to spring into action; cold extremities, as essential blood supplies are directed to the brain, muscles and lungs; and becoming more alert and our senses sharpening by the action of increased levels of noradrenaline, thus our sense of hearing, smell, touch and sight become more acute. People under extreme and acute stress often claim their vision becomes blurred and they are sensitive to noise levels when under stress. Table 1.2 provides a detailed list of the physical, emotional and behavioural signs of distress.

Stress and the stress response, in an evolutionary sense, are good for us and have been necessary for the

Table 1.2   Signs of distress

Physical indicators
- Aware of heart beating, palpitations and chest pains; dizziness
- Breathlessness – breathing difficulties (hyperventilation); rapid shallow breathing
- Dry mouth; feeling 'a lump in the throat'; 'butterflies' in stomach, indigestion, nausea; cramps
- Tingling in muscles – particularly the arms and legs
- Eyelid or facial muscle twitch; over-sensitive to noise
- General muscle tenseness – particularly of the jaws; grinding of teeth; clenched fists; hunched shoulders
- General muscle aches, pains and cramps; migraine, headache
- Sweaty – especially the palms and upper lip, hot flushed feeling; cold fingers and toes
- Changes in menstrual patterns; impotence

Mental or emotional signs (covert signs of stress)
- Distressed, worried and feeling unable to cope
- Feeling neglected, insecure and vulnerable; worrying unreasonably about things; feelings of helplessness
- Frustrated; bored; inadequate; guilt; panic
- Excessive and rapid swings of mood
- Wanting to withdraw into daydreams
- Feeling tired all the time; lack of concentration
- Irritable, impatient – response internalized
- Anxious; depressed; excessive concerns about physical health
- Inability to feel sympathy for other people; apathy
- Pent-up anger

Behavioural signs of stress (overt signs)
- Tearful – emotional response to minor issues
- Aggression; hostility and irritability towards other people; overreactive; loss of control
- Indecision; procrastination
- Having so much to do and not knowing where to start so ending up doing nothing; or going from task to task and not completing anything, i.e. polyphasic behaviour – doing many things at once – always rushed
- Unreasonable complaints; hypercritical; inflexible
- Non-productive; poor job performance; inefficient
- Resistant to change – clings to familiar routine; obsessional behaviours; lack of creativity
- Vulnerable to accidents; careless driving; prone to mistakes
- TATT (tired all the time); sleep problems; looks sick
- Lack of interest in sport, hobbies and leisure pursuits

Table 1.2 *continued*

- Lack of interest in self-appearance; loss of libido; change in eating habits – skipping meals, bingeing
- Bite nails – twist hair
- Increase in use of cigarettes or alcohol; drug dependence – including caffeine
- Delayed recovery from illness or accidents
- Lying or cheating to 'cover-up'

development of our society. It has been described as an adaptation for life on the savannah and our response to stress was meant to be both adaptive and vital for survival. In the past we had simple choices to make. Either stand and fight an enemy, or run away from a threatening and potentially dangerous situation. However, in contemporary society and medical practice, medical practitioners face a dilemma because neither of these options is appropriate behaviour in a hospital environment or practice clinic. Typically in the work environment of the medical practitioner there is little opportunity to indulge in the level of physical action needed to dissipate the physiological effects that become dominant and can cause distress. Indeed, that natural response to stress is denied, since the doctor cannot physically fight to escape workplace stress, and neither is it an option to turn around and run away from a situation. At such times the body remains primed to take actions that are denied. Many doctors also lead increasingly sedentary lives at work and at home, and they, just like many of their patients, are unable to release the aggression by engaging in the physical activity necessary to effectively remove the build up of hormones resulting from exposure to stress.

As one GP observed,

I have measured my blood pressure at the beginning and the end of surgery. It can be normal at the start (135/85) and up to 185/100 at the end. This is especially true when I find myself running late. Nevertheless, denial of the existence of stress is still commonly observed because only people who are not up to the job feel like that.

Whilst our response to stress is in the first instance physiological, it is recognized that complex emotional and behavioural reactions are involved (see Table 1.2). These can lead to potentially damaging health outcomes. Understanding the nature of stress in these terms helps us to think positively and pro-actively about stress instead of taking a defensive, self-blaming stance. We are all exposed to potentially stressful situations and are, therefore, vulnerable. However, the way in which we handle stress can magnify the problem and be the cause of many physical ill health problems. We describe this as coping by using maladaptive strategies.

Adaptive versus maladaptive ways of coping with stress

Coping is described as the cognitive and behavioural efforts made to meet demands perceived as exceeding our personal resources (Lazarus & Folkman 1984). A distinction is made between coping that is perceived as adaptive and that which is described as maladaptive (Cooper et al. 1988). This is the basis of our assumption that stress is inevitable, but that it is mismanaged stress that is damaging in its consequences. Therefore, there is a need for doctors to manage potentially stressful situations in a proactive and positive manner rather than resorting to maladaptive ways of coping. Maladaptive usually refers to coping strategies that are primarily avoidance of the problem (Spurgeon et al. 1997). Such strategies are unlikely to result in long-term solutions and, typically, will lead to additional stress, and concomitant health and behaviour problems. Maladaptive coping strategies include:

1. An excessive use of alcohol or nicotine: Shaffer (1983) states that smoking cigarettes is viewed as a pick-me-up or social activity that also provides energy, but it also causes indigestion and poor sleep; drinking alcohol is a social activity and muscle relaxant, but is also a depressant and energy drain.

2. Substance abuse and dependence drugs, including tranquillisers, sleeping pills, 'pep' pills and caffeine.
3. The couch potato syndrome: a lack of physical activity when not working, usually as a result of being tired all the time. Thus the individual fails to take adequate levels of physical activity and exercise, or engage in fulfilling social and recreational activities.
4. Eat more, eat less, or engage in comfort eating when we feel sorry for ourselves; the problem is exacerbated when we binge on foods high in sugars and fats, and which have empty calories, and low or poor nutritional value; eating sugar or chocolate is seen as a pick-me-up, but they are only empty calories (Shaffer 1983).
5. Procrastination: when we feel stressed we often put off dealing with a situation, or try not to think about it because it is threatening or too difficult. Whilst there might be a case for doing nothing on some occasions, it is likely that stress problems tend to escalate if avoided and appropriate action is delayed. This usually results in the creation of greater and more difficult problems to tackle. Sleeping on a problem can often help the individual to identify a solution to a difficult situation; however, a night of disturbed and troubled sleep caused by worry and an inability or unwillingness to confront a problem is a maladaptive way of coping with the stressful situation. It also renders the individual less able to cope with a problem the following day.
6. Becoming angry and aggressive with ourselves and other people. This is a particularly damaging strategy if we persist in internalizing by keeping our feelings to ourself or 'bottling our anger up'. This quietly seething time bomb becomes dangerous and unstable and might cause irreparable damage when a subsequent, and often minor or insignificant event, finally leads to a major 'explosion'.

Research evidence suggests coping style is an important variable in the stress-management process. For example, use of social support as a coping strategy has a positive effect on mental health (Cohen et al. 1985), and among a sample of UK GPs it was found to be significantly associated with reported job-satisfaction levels (Sutherland & Cooper 1993). Coping using emotion-focused strategies is often associated with poorer mental health (Edwards & Baglioni 1990). Hospital consultants in Scotland with a high level of burnout tended to cope with job stress by expressing high levels of negative emotion (Deary et al. 1996). In a study of Swiss dentists, Heim (1991) found that the use of support from both work and social relationships, tackling problems directly and the use of humour were associated with professional satisfaction. Denial of problems, being resigned to a stressful situation, social withdrawal and the consumption of above average amounts of alcohol or drugs was associated with job dissatisfaction among this professional group. Likewise, hospital doctors who used avoidance, or wishful thinking, when experiencing stress at work were found to have poorer mental health than those who did not adopt such passive strategies (Tattersall et al. 1999). In a large-scale study of hospital consultants, Graham et al. (2001) observed that the consultants who reported using alcohol or non-prescriptive drugs in response to stress were more than twice as likely to experience psychiatric morbidity as those who maintained a balanced, healthy lifestyle while experiencing stress at work. In this survey, the 882 consultants (out of a population of 1133) reported that they coped with stress by:

- talking to a partner, family or friends – 70%
- talking to colleagues informally – 67%
- working longer hours – 53%
- pursuing hobbies or leisure activities – 51%
- taking annual leave – 39%
- taking exercise or playing sport – 36%
- drinking alcohol – 26%
- not eating as healthily as you would wish – 24%
- reorganizing your work to reduce stress – 19%
- talking to colleagues, formally in a regular support group – 12%

- learning techniques for relaxation – 4%
- smoking cigarettes – 3%
- taking prescription drugs – 3%
- obtaining formal psychological support – 2%
- taking other (non-prescription) drugs – 0.5%

Quite clearly, this study shows that there are large numbers of hospital consultants using maladaptive ways of coping with stress to the detriment of their own health. The impact of this behaviour on their job performance was not examined. Cross-sectional studies of this nature do not help us to understand the issue of causation, i.e. what came first, the alcohol and drugs, or the stress? However, enough evidence exists to indicate that maladaptive coping strategies are dangerous because they can render us less fit to cope with the demands of work, and in the long term can actually become a source of stress themself when, for example, addiction or ill health escalates. The topic of maladaptive coping is discussed further in the final chapter.

Change as a source of stress

The rate of change for professionals working in the medical health services has been rapid and unrelenting. For the past 20 years in the UK the government's drive to increase efficiency and the concomitant changes have created a more turbulent, commercial environment, much dissatisfaction and an increase in doctors' workloads (British Medical Association 1992, Hannay et al. 1992; Sutherland & Cooper 1992, Swanson & Power 1996). In Canada, the conflict relationship between the medical profession and government, and the resulting militant action and activities was caused by unwanted government intrusion and pressure to control healthcare costs. Changes stemmed from the introduction of universal government health insurance in the 1960s (Touhy 1976, Stevenson & Williams 1985) and caused physicians to try to defend their professional autonomy, ultimately by a strike in 1970 among Quebec specialists. This situation remained unresolved and a lengthy period of tension followed. It culminated in the Ontario doctors' strike of 1986, which resulted in the withdrawal of all but emergency services for a period of 25 days.

Research evidence indicates that a wide variety of workplace conditions cause stress, strain or pressure and are associated with physical and psychological health problems. However, change and the changing nature of the work environment can be a potent source of stress and pressure. Response to change must be dealt with in a positive way if the doctor is to remain healthy and successful as a carer for other people. As we have observed, constant change has been the dominant theme in the health service in the latter part of the 20th century and this pattern seems set to continue into this millennium. While doctors endeavour to meet the demands associated with predictable life-event changes, they must continue to face the endless re-shaping of their work structure and climate, the changing nature of society, and the concomitant demands of life in the new millennium. Change, it is said, brings about progress and improvement to our quality of life. It can provide stimulation, variety and relief from boredom. Indeed, why would we wish to make changes for the worse? It is suggested that problems arise because the medical practice work environment has become a place of rapid, discontinuous change that requires us to live in a state of transience and impermanence. The situation is potentially damaging because energy is needed for and expended by the constant adaptation to the external environment. Whether we welcome, fear or resist change, adaptation and adjustment requires energy. Thus, it is said that change is not made without inconvenience, even change for the better.

Hans Selye (1976) reminds us that the energy resources needed to implement change are not infinite and so breakdown of the system, in part or total, will ultimately occur. In Selye's view, impairment of function and structural change are wholly, or in part, linked to adaptation to stimulation or 'arousal'. Exposure to a continued state of arousal will result in wear and tear on the body. This chemical wear and tear on the body is defined as the ageing process, which in the extreme can lead to exhaustion, collapse and ultimately early death. A cynic might suggest that change is to be expected from everything except vending machines! Clearly change is here to stay, and this old adage is a truth that permeates all our lives (Cooper et al. 1988). Exposure to 'change' as a source of stress is an inevitable part of modern-day living and working for the doctor, and unless it is effectively managed this form of workplace stress can result in adverse and costly outcomes for both doctor and patient.

A transactional model of stress

In summary, we suggest that stress can be viewed as a condition, a response to an event, or the event itself. Bailey and Clark (1989) propose three approaches to the understanding of stress:

- The stimulus-based model of stress where stress is viewed as something external to the doctor, to which there is a reaction. For example, a patient who fails to keep an appointment, or behaves in an abusive manner is a source of stress (or stressor) and the doctor reacts by experiencing strain or pressure. The weakness of this approach is that it treats 'the doctor' as a passive respondent to a stress event, whereas in reality there are many factors that might mediate the outcome in such a situation.
- The response-based approach to stress, in which the focus of attention is the doctors' physiological, psychological or behavioural response to a stress situation. This approach to stress management is mainly concerned with dealing with symptoms of stress.
- Finally, the approach that involves regarding the stress process as a transaction between the environment and the doctor. Both of the above approaches have many

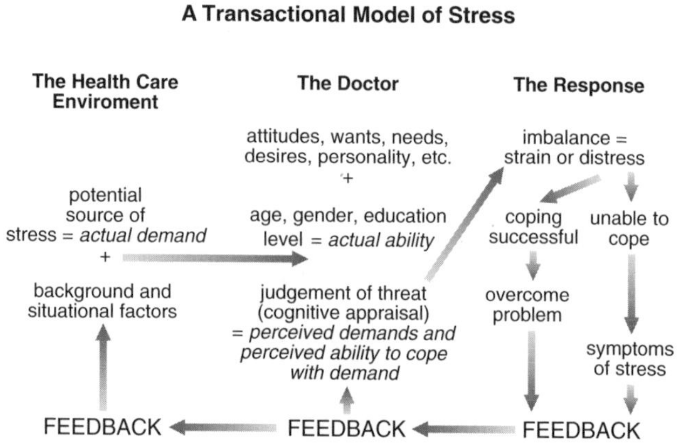

A Transactional Model of Stress

The Health Care Enviroment	The Doctor	The Response

attitudes, wants, needs, desires, personality, etc.
+
age, gender, education level = *actual ability*

potential source of stress = *actual demand*
+
background and situational factors

judgement of threat (cognitive appraisal) = *perceived demands and perceived ability to cope with demand*

imbalance = strain or distress

coping successful   unable to cope

overcome problem

symptoms of stress

FEEDBACK ◄━━━ FEEDBACK ◄━━━ FEEDBACK

Figure 1.2   A Transactional Model of Stress

inherent weaknesses, and so this approach is more useful (see Figure 1.2).

Therefore, we will be using the transactional model to understand and explain the stress process. This model has five key provisos that have important implications for the process and effective management of stress: These include:

1. The notion that 'stress is not simply out there in the environment'. A situation has to be perceived as a source of stress in order to be so. Since we cognitively appraise the situation, stress is a subjective experience contingent upon the perception of an event – it is a perceived demand. As Shakespeare's 'Hamlet', says, 'There is nothing good or bad, but thinking makes it so'.

2. The way a situation or event is perceived depends upon familiarity with the situation, previous exposure to the event, learning, education and training, etc. Experience shapes an individual's perceived ability to cope with a threat or demand.

3. Pressure or stress is the mismatch between demands – that is, actual demand, perceived demand, actual ability and perceived ability. Needs, desires and the level of arousal will influence the way in which a potential source of stress is perceived. A state of stress will exist

either because we have wrongly judged the situation, or our ability to deal with it. Stress management teaches us to overcome this form of 'faulty thinking'

4. A potential source of stress is not perceived in a social vacuum. The presence or absence of other doctors or work colleagues will affect our perception of a potentially stressful situation – this is described as an 'interpersonal influence'. In a stressful situation we tend to look at the behaviour of the people around us if we are unsure how to behave or interpret the situation. We seek cues and act upon them whilst also taking into account the status or experience of these significant and important others.

5. A state of stress is acknowledged as an imbalance or mismatch between the perceived 'demand' and the perception of one's ability to meet that demand. The processes that follow are the coping process and the consequences of the coping strategy applied. Successful coping restores balance, but unsuccessful coping results in the manifestation of symptoms of exposure to stress. The response may produce short-term reactions, in the form of maladaptive coping strategies such as, 'light another cigarette', 'need alcohol' or 'take a sleeping pill'; or it may ultimately result in long-term effects such as heart disease, certain forms of cancer or ulcers. Therefore, it is acknowledged that the short-term consequences of exposure to stress and maladaptive coping strategies can also be causal factors in the aetiology of certain long-term diseases and illness (for example, the link between cigarette smoking and alcohol consumption, and the incidence of lung cancer and diseases of the liver). Thus, a method of coping with a source of stress can ultimately become the source of stress itself!

A transactional process model of stress acknowledges that situations are not inherently stressful, but are potentially stressful, and it is necessary to take account of the:

• environment in which the source of stress exists
• source of stress, known as the 'stressor' or stress agent

- individual differences that moderate or mediate in our response to stress
- stress response; that is the physical, emotional, or behavioural outcomes of exposure to stress.

These are discussed further in the next chapter, on stress diagnosis or analysis.

Defining stress

Therefore, our understanding of stress must be in terms of a transactional process model. Stress is a dynamic condition in which time plays a vital role. There are many definitions of stress, and it might be simply said that 'stress is unwanted pressure'. However, Beehr and Newman (1978) provide us with a comprehensive definition of job stress that also guides our stress identification and stress-management processes. They state that stress is, ' . . . . a situation wherein job-related factors interact with a worker to change (that is, disrupt or enhance) his or her psychological and or physiological condition such that the person (that is, mind or body) is forced to deviate from normal functioning. This definition also serves to define what we mean by 'employee health'; namely a person's mental and physical condition. We are referring to health in its broadest sense – the complete continuum from superb mental and physical health all the way to death. Note, that we are not excluding the possibility of beneficial effects of stress on health'.

Accepting this definition permits us to agree with Hans Selye's view that the only person without stress is a dead person. In reality we are not in the position to test his hypothesis and, of course, are happy not to do so! We accept the position that stress is stimulation, challenge, variety and the spice of life – stress is inevitable – distress is not! Nevertheless, mismanaged stress and unwanted pressure is damaging in its consequences. In the next chapter we consider practical ways of identifying stress.

chapter TWO

Stress diagnosis

In Chapter one we argued that stress management (ACTION) is successful only when it is based on a firm understanding of the stress process (AWARENESS) and a method of identifying the source of stress (ANALYSIS). It is also suggested that we should tackle stress at three levels and so the following tripartite model of stress management is recommended.

- LEVEL ONE – To prevent or minimize the stress of medical practice where this is possible and reasonably practicable. This is known as primary level stress management.
- LEVEL TWO – To assist individual doctors, teams or groups in general practice or hospitals, through education and training, to cope more effectively with stress that cannot be eliminated or minimized. This is known as secondary level stress management.
- LEVEL THREE – To have in place strategies to deal with doctors and their staff who 'fall through the net' to become victims of exposure to stress, since no intervention is likely to be perfect or foolproof. As individuals, we are complex and unique and vary in our response to stress and so a stress-management solution for one doctor will not suit or benefit all. This curative approach to stress management is known as tertiary care.

In order to take the best course of action it is necessary to identify the source of stress. This chapter offers practical ways of diagnosing stress. In formal terms this process is described as a stress audit or psychological risk assessment. A model for the stress audit process is described next to enable the doctor, as a manager of other people, to identify the stress that exists in a practice business or hospital clinic, department or section. It also includes guidelines for the individual doctor in the identification of stress.

The stress audit

Any situation or event is potentially stressful and so it is necessary to distinguish between positive and negative pressures in the work environment of the doctor. Thus, it is important to identify the barriers to both job performance and well-being by asking, 'what, who, where, why, when and how?' This is the essence of a 'stress audit' and it should be conducted in a systematic and objective way. Stress audits are used to identify individual and organizational strengths and weaknesses, and so can be compared in many ways to a training, or development needs analysis. At a more informal level it might also be described in terms of a 'SWOT' analysis. By this process each individual, or a team of doctors, can identify the 'strengths, weakness, opportunities and threats' inherent in the job, and use the information to decide on a course of remedial action.

The stress audit process is used to understand work stress problems and the attitudes of doctors and their staff towards both the perceived problems and the possible solutions. Involvement and participation are an essential part of this process, which helps to overcome any resistance to the changes associated with the subsequent introduction of stress-management initiatives. It will also help to reduce the threat or fear associated with potentially sensitive stress-related issues in the medical practice work environment.

Components of a stress audit

Essentially, there are five key components in the stress audit process (see Figure 2.1)

1. Measure sources of stress. We need to identify and measure the sources of stress that exist. The model of stress proposed by Cooper and Marshall (1978) conceptualizes stress within six main categories, described as:

   a. factors intrinsic to the job – for example, patient overload and excessive job demands; time pressures; administrative overload and practice administration; unpredictable interruptions/telephone interruptions; disruptive events; inadequate time for preparation; inadequate resources and staff; long waiting lists.

   b. one's role in the organization – for example, role-related demand; dealing with death and dying; emotional involvement and demand; confrontation with emotional suffering; feelings of helplessness

   c. relationships with other people – for example, staff conflicts; stress among colleagues; patients' unrealistic expectations and demands; coping with difficult patients; inexperienced personnel; physical or verbal assault

   d. career development and achievement – for example, professional development; threat of malpractice suits

   e. organizational structure and climate, that is, the culture and climate of the practice, hospital or health organization – for example, strict regulations; loss of autonomy and lack of personal control

   f. the home–work interface – for example, stress overspill from work to home and vice versa; family–job conflicts; disruptions to social life; lack of leisure and free time; demands of work on family time.

   Use these categories as a guide in the identification of sources of stress within your group or team.

2. Measure stress outcomes. This means the measurement of performance indicators and might include such things as patient complaints; mistakes made by the doctor or staff; poor performance, such as the loss of medical records or the results of medical tests, or work not completed on time. In business terms, measures

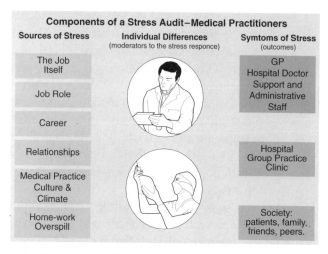

Components of a Stress Audit–Medical Practitioners

Figure 2.1   Components of a Stress Audit – medical practitioners

such as days lost due to ill health, physical symptoms of ill health, accidents at work, job dissatisfaction levels, labour turnover or staff grievances may be used. It is also possible to measure emotional state, such as levels of anxiety or depression, as symptoms of exposure to stress.

3. Measure individual differences. Acknowledge and identify the individual differences that moderate our response to stress. Typically these include a wide variety of individual differences that act to shape our response to exposure to stress and must be taken into account when understanding stress. These include:

    a. physical condition, such as levels of fitness and health, life stage, diet and eating habits, exercise activity, sleep patterns, relaxation activities, hobbies or interests

    b. biographic and demographic differences, such as age, gender, race, occupation, education and training, and socio-economic status.

    c. personality traits and behavioural characteristics, for example, extroversion, neuroticism, need for achievement and power, Type A behaviour, and the need for control, i.e. Locus of Control, etc.

4. Identify stress predictors. Identify the sources of stress most closely associated with the outcomes measured. For example, in the audit conducted among GPs in the UK (Sutherland 1995) it was observed that the predictors of high levels of depression were:
   a. high levels of demand in the job itself and patient expectations of the doctors
   b. the stress associated with trying to balance work and home life demands
   c. low use of social support as a strategy for coping with stress.

Therefore, the strategies recommended for stress control among GPs were to:

   i. initiate a campaign to educate the public about the role of the general practitioner, particularly with respect to night calls and locum duties
   ii. make optimal use of support staff; delegate tasks where possible; re-examine time-management skills
   iii. increase levels of social support by having regular meetings out of surgery hours and extending the sessions into social gatherings to include partners and spouses.

5. Understand doctor and staff attitudes to the options available for the management of stress. That is, acknowledge and understand what doctors (and practice and medical support staff) need and want in place in order to remove the stressor barriers to their effectiveness, productivity, health and job satisfaction.

The process of stress diagnosis

A wide variety of techniques and methods are available in the stress diagnosis process. These include:

- stress logs or diaries – useful for the individual doctor as an aid to stress diagnosis
- critical-incident techniques – can be used at an individual or group level

- focus-group sessions – useful for the hospital team, department, clinic or surgery practice
- one-to-one or group interviews – also used by the doctor in a managerial or supervisory capacity
- work-related records – a variety of business records can help in the diagnosis of a potential stress problem
- questionnaires – these can be used on an individual or group basis.

Using a stress log to identify stress

Each day, the doctor records the most stressful experience(s) of the day, what happened, what they did in the situation, the people involved, the feelings or reactions experienced and, on reflection, what they might have done differently (see Appendix I). The diary should include both work-and home-related experiences. By accumulating this information over a period of time it is possible to observe re-occurring patterns of stressful experiences, the need for action and the type of action required to resolve the problem. Usually a 7-day period of log keeping is needed initially, but this depends upon the work schedule and routine of the individual. A group or team can also keep logs or diaries, and then exchange and discuss the information in a group-discussion session. By collating this information it is possible to identify the key sources of stress among the group and agree suitable action strategies to overcome the problems identified.

Using 'critical-incident' analysis to identify stress

Critical-incident analysis is used in interview and focus-group sessions to identify potential sources of stress. The doctor or team is asked to describe job-related events that they believe have created difficult or unmet demands, and thereby caused difficulties resulting in a negative impact on job performance or personal well-being. It is important to try to remain specific and non-emotive about the incident. For example, 'misplaced a patient's record – felt upset and angry all day' is too general a description of stress and is not specific enough. Whilst it is useful to acknowledge emotion, it is important to objectively identify the cause of the problem because it is likely to also point to a solution to the stress problem. For example, 'My day was disrupted because I wasted valuable time chasing a patient's record; I was tired last night so did not ensure that I was prepared for the early morning duty; I got up late and so did not allow myself adequate time to make certain that everything was ready for the early start'. This is a specific and non-emotive description of the event. It assists the individual in finding ways to eliminate this particular source of stress in the future by ensuring that time-management and delegation skills are used. Clearly, a negative reaction is one that results in an argument with support staff or feeling angry with yourself, or other people. Continuing to behave in a disruptive manner for the remainder of the day is likely to be harmful in the long term. In the final stage of the critical-incident process, the individual or group is asked how they felt about the consequences of their behaviour in response to the situation.

Often an external agent guides and monitors this process. It is important that a facilitator or interviewer does not judge or evaluate the situation or the response. Critical-incident analysis will reveal specific stressors, behaviours and consequences, in addition to coping style trends and preferences. The technique can be successfully applied to identify key sources of stress among a particular work group or team, or for a specific individual.

Using a focus group to identify stress

It is possible for a small group of doctors, doctors and their practice, or departmental staff to meet and use brainstorming techniques to identify the source(s) of stress that exist and act as barriers to their performance effectiveness, job satisfaction and quality of work life. Typically, a facilitator acts as an independent observer and communicator for the focus group, but a group of doctors acting independently, who understand the rules of conducting a focus-group session, can use this technique. Usually the group will complete individual stress logs or diaries for a week before the session and use this information to maximize the time spent in the group session. It is suggested that some preparation is done in advance to start the thinking process. We recommend, as a minimum, that each person completes a pro-forma that asks questions such as:

- What is the best thing about the job?
- What is the worst thing about the job?
- What advice would you give to a new colleague?
- What advice would you give to a son or daughter going into medical practice?

or:

- What are the strongest barriers to your performance effectiveness as a doctor (practice nurse or receptionist etc.)?
- What are the strongest facilitators of your performance effectiveness as a doctor (practice nurse or receptionist etc.)?
- If you had the fairy godmother's wand, what would you change (in the surgery, the hospital team, the practice or clinic etc.) to improve your performance effectiveness as a doctor (practice nurse or receptionist)?
- Do you believe that you have a good balance between your work and home-life? If the answer is 'no', what can be done to improve this situation?
    - by you personally
    - by your team or group
    - by the system (e.g. hospital management, medical association, government/legislative levels).

Using interviews to identify stress

One-to-one or group interviews can be used to identify sources of stress in medical practice. The unique and confidential nature of stress-related problems and the sensitive issues involved often make this a preferred option in the identification of potential stressors. However, whilst it is possible that a doctor might conduct an interview with a member of staff, it is also likely that the interview process will be in the hands of an external consultant or trained counsellor if the doctor is also the first-line manager of the person concerned. The interview process may be combined with some of the techniques already described above, however, the success of the method depends upon the skills of the interviewer. Interviewing and the analysis of the interview materials are time-consuming processes, subject to the errors inherent in this technique. The need for sensitivity and caution is paramount.

Using work records to identify stress

Information from existing work records can be used to support the findings from self-report information obtained from interviews, questionnaires, stress logs or a critical-incident analysis. These might include, for example, sickness absence records, grievance records and patient complaints, patient satisfaction data, or the cost of compensation claims or malpractice suits. However, Rees (1995) found that hospital doctors did not seem to be taking sickness absence resulting from stress, compared with other hospital staff and so these records are unlikely to be helpful. More importantly, he suggests that this is probably an indication that stressed doctors continue to work while highly stressed.

Using questionnaires to identify stress

A variety of standardized measures are available to identify and measure stress and these have the advantage of providing normative data comparisons. Whilst many questionnaires are 'paper and pencil' instruments, the use of computerized assessment has simplified the procedure considerably. One extensively used instrument in the UK is the Occupational Stress Indicator (OSI) devised by Cooper et al. (1988). This questionnaire is a comprehensive package that adopts the model of stress proposed by Cooper and Marshall (1978). It is possible to obtain individual stress profiles, and group or team profiles, in addition to large sample data results with normative comparisons. The OSI includes measures such as:

- sources of stress – stress is measured according to the six factors already described above (see Figure 2.1)
- mental and physical well-being
- job satisfaction levels
- stress coping styles, such as time management and use of social support
- personality and behavioural style (Type A behaviour and Locus of Control).

Other instruments can be used to measure single variables, such as the Crown Crisp Experiential Index (CCEI) (Crown & Crisp 1979) for the measurement of mental health, or the measurement of job satisfaction developed by Warr et al. (1979).

However, we suggest that a standardized questionnaire is not able to include all the sources of stress unique to particular occupations. Therefore, a stressor item bank unique to the group should be generated from the stress log or focus-group information. The case study of stress among GPs described below illustrates this process. Some questionnaires are tailored specifically to meet the needs of a project. For example, the study to understand physician militancy in Canada (Burke 2001) used a seven-page self-administered questionnaire comprising of:

- work experiences – hours worked, complaints against health insurance bureaucracies, problem patients (e.g. patients insisting on hospitalization, failure to comply with instructions), perceptions of increased workload
- gender
- level of stress – how stressful medical practice was perceived to be
- work satisfaction – level of satisfaction in the practice of medicine under Medicare
- physician militancy – attitudes to the reconstitution of medical associations as labour unions under provincial labour laws and attitude to withdrawal of services by

physicians if negotiations with government fail to produce satisfactory settlement.

It can be seen that the scope for stress audit and analysis is very broad and without limits. Ultimately any questionnaire must be valid, reliable, credible and acceptable to the respondents. Ethical issues concerning the use of data and confidentiality must be adhered to and respected. This leads us to the consideration of who should be involved in implementation of a stress audit.

Who does the stress audit?

Audits conducted by personnel internal to a practice, hospital or clinic, gain benefit because those who know the business are managing the stress audit process. Unfortunately, it also means that the findings can become distorted. This is usually not intentional, but an artefact of the process and caused by the pre-conceived notions of the individuals involved. On a practical note, we must also consider whether internal personnel, tasked with the audit, fulfil the following requirements.

1. Do they have the time to conduct a stress audit project?
2. Do they have the appropriate skills and qualifications?
3. Can they be objective and remain discreet in order to guarantee anonymity and confidentiality?
4. Is there likely to be any risk of breach of ethics?
5. Do they have the trust and respect of the staff that are being audited?
6. Is it possible that influence, either direct or indirect, from other stakeholders or 'politicians' within the practice or hospital setting could affect the findings? Pressure from powerful (or feared) others can result in information being withheld, omitted or distorted, thereby corrupting the results of the stress audit or risk assessment.

The use of an external body to conduct the stress audit will overcome many of the concerns expressed above, particularly those associated with the issues of objectivity and confidentiality. However, these outsiders will know little about the business initially and will need to spend time becoming familiar with the culture and climate of the hospital or practice. It is also likely that the costs will be higher. Whilst the use of computers for the administration, scoring and interpretation of audit instruments has helped business managers to be self-sufficient in the stress audit process, many still prefer to use the help of external agencies in a nominal way in order to add credibility and objectivity to the audit exercise. If the audit is on a large scale, the data analysis can be a lengthy procedure since the results should identify sub-group differences, for example, between job specialization, department, job grade, and type of contract (i.e. full- or part-time working). Also, to take into account factors of gender, age, length of service, and medical setting, etc. This will ensure that stress control actions are targeted specifically where needed in order to be successful and cost effective.

We have already advised that it is important to identify data already available within the practice, clinic or hospital and to integrate this into the risk-assessment process. Ideally, a stress audit should not be a 'stand-alone' exercise. Indeed, it is also worth considering whether the term 'stress audit' is to be used. Since the word stress still has negative connotations, it means that a 'stress audit' is often perceived as a threat to those taking part in the process. If doctors and staff greet the audit with suspicion and suspect some other 'real' purpose, they will feel threatened and unlikely to co-operate. They might also feel that they are being blamed for not coping with stress and may try to overcome this by denying that any stress-related problems exist. Typically, in this situation, people try to behave like swans, gliding serenely on the surface of a smooth lake, appearing to be calm and in control. However, just like a swan, all the frantic activity remains hidden beneath the surface! Ultimately, the objective of a stress audit is to optimize the job performance and health (that is, the work–life balance and well-being) of doctors and staff, so why not describe it as such, and avoid using the word stress in such a high profile and potentially threatening way? In the final section of this chapter we describe a stress audit conducted among general practitioners, and provide a brief description of the findings and the recommendations.

A stress-audit case study: to identify ill health and job dissatisfaction among GPs working in the UK

The objective of this audit was to identify the sources of job stress and the personality factors that were most predictive of psychological ill health and job dissatisfaction among GPs working in the UK (Sutherland & Cooper 1992). The investigation followed enforced changes to the ways of working and contractual arrangements, which resulted in reports of increased pressure at work for GPs. Much of this had been caused by financial constraints, the needs of ever demanding patients, increasing practice administration duties and an element of uncertainty. A four-phased approach was required in order to identify negative stress.

1. To identify stressors in the unique work environment of the GP.
2. To examine certain individual mediators of the stress response.
3. To measure the well-being of GPs in terms of certain known manifestations of exposure to stress, including psychological ill health, job dissatisfaction and the use of maladaptive coping mechanisms (e.g alcohol and drug abuse).
4. To identify the stressors most strongly associated with negative outcomes – that is, job dissatisfaction, depression and anxiety – and the possible causes of stress-related health problems.

Following a series of focus-group sessions with a geographic, stratified sample of GPs, a questionnaire was designed for distribution to a national sample. The questionnaire was sent to a randomly selected group of 1500 GPs. A guarantee of confidentiality was given. Sources of stress were measured in two ways: a 31-stressor item bank developed from interviews conducted by Cooper et al. (1989) was used together with the sources of a job pressure scale from the OSI. Some general information gleaned from the survey included:

- 917 GPs took part in the survey
- 670 male and 243 female doctors
- most GPs were working in a group practice (93%) and were working from one (69%) or two (25%) surgeries
- only 27 of the GP respondents worked part-time.

Audit results

In this section a brief account of the audit findings are described. Table 2.1 shows the sources of stress identified by this group of GPs classified as stressor factors. The research findings indicated that the male GPs were found to be significantly more anxious and depressed compared with a British normative sample of men, whereas the observed scores for the women doctors were similar to the population norms for women.

The main predictors of job dissatisfaction among GPs were:

1. pressure associated with the demands of the job and patients' expectations (see Table 2.1)
2. the stress of the organization structure and climate, and the home and work interface (see Table 2.1)
3. low use of social support as a coping strategy, although women doctors were more likely to use social support as a method of coping than the male GPs
4. GPs who practised from more than one surgery were most likely to be dissatisfied with the job, and job satisfaction levels decreased as the number of practice premises increased.

High levels of anxiety were associated with job-role stress, the demands of the job and the high expectations

Table 2.1 Stress factors and stressor items for GPs

Factor 1. Demands of job and patients' expectations
Fear of assault during night visits
Visiting in extremely adverse weather conditions
Adverse publicity by media
Increased demand by patients and relatives for second opinion from hospital specialists
No appreciation of your work by patients
Worrying about patients' complaints
Finding a locum
Twenty-four hour responsibility for patients' lives
Taking several samples in a short time
Unrealistically high expectations by others of your role

Factor 2. Interruptions
Coping with phone calls during night and early morning
Night calls
Interruption of family life by telephone
Emergency calls during surgery hours
Home visits
Dealing with problem patients
Remaining alert when on call

Factor 3. Practice administration and routine medical
Hospital referrals and paperwork
Conducting surgery
Practice administration
Arranging admissions
Working environment (surgery set-up)
Time pressure

Factor 4. Home-work interface and social life
Demands of your job on family life
Dividing time between your spouse and patients
Demands of job on social life
Lack of emotional support at home, especially from spouse

Factor 5. Dealing with death and dying
Daily contact with dying and chronically ill patients
Dealing with the terminally ill and their relatives

Factor 6. Medical responsibility for friends and relatives
Dealing with friends as patients
Dealing with relatives as patients

Cited by Cooper et al. (1989)

of their patients, and the stress of practice administration and routine medical work. No differences were observed between the male and female doctors. Doctors who exhibited the Type A coronary-prone style of behaviour were also more likely to exhibit higher levels of anxiety than their Type B colleagues. Doctors who operated from more than one surgery were also more likely to exhibit higher levels of anxiety.

High levels of depression were related to the demands of the job, the high expectations of their patients, and the stress of the home and work interface. Low use of social support as a source of coping was also associated with high levels of depression.

Therefore, four main themes appear to emerge from this stress audit.

1. The pressures of the demands of the job and patients' expectations were key sources of stress. This included the increasing fear of assault during night visits, worry about complaints from patients, the high expectations of patients and adverse publicity by the media. Doctors felt that their patients had not been fully informed about the changes necessary for them to fulfil the terms of the new contract and this caused needless conflict between doctor and patient, especially for call-out arrangements.

2. Role stress appeared to be associated with poor psychological well-being. Not surprising, in the aftermath of so much change, these pressures were due to conflict between the job task and the new role demands on GPs. Role ambiguity, the implications of making mistakes, and being highly visible were key sources of stress. GPs reported that they no longer felt in control of the events that affected their ways of working and did not feel that they were adequately consulted about the changes made to their job and way of life as a GP.

3. The third key stressor could be characterized as 'being in the organization', and describes the work structure and climate of the GP. These sources of stress included,

a lack of consultation and communication, having to do mundane administrative work, having insufficient resources to do the job effectively, staff shortages, lack of feedback about one's performance and low morale. Essentially, many GPs did not like working in large group-practice environments, which by necessity were usually run by a business practice manager.

4. The role of social support was a contributory factor in the well-being of the general practitioner and was a significant predictor of both job satisfaction levels and depression. Since women doctors were more likely to report using social support as a stress-coping strategy, and exhibited a better level of psychological well-being and job satisfaction than the male doctors, this was recommended as an area worthy of more investigation as a stress-management technique among doctors.

Audit recommendations

In addition to an increased awareness of individual strategies to improve personal fitness for coping with stress, such as relaxation, increased physical activity/exercise, time-management or assertion training, suggestions for stress control at the group and business level included:

1. Team development and team building, and interpersonal skills training as a way of helping to alleviate or eliminate stress in the group-practice work environment of the GPs. Crucial, however, were opportunities to build support networks and to allocate work appropriately. Both partnership and staff relationship problems could be addressed by more effective team working.

2. At the highest level, in organizational terms, stress management would operate by seeking to eliminate or minimize problems identified by the GPs. This was at the level of the NHS, where the general-practice model could be examined in consultation with those working in general practice. It was apparent that GPs believed that they needed to be more involved in the decisions

and actions that affected them. The concept of team management could be used to examine models of job design, methods of working and the use of new technology to reduce the administrative demands on the GP.

3. Stress-management strategies to include the provision of equipment to improve the safety of doctors on call, such as mobile phones, radio alarms and car alarms.

4. Importantly, it was felt that stress levels could be reduced if a message was communicated to patients, about the need for more realistic expectations of the GP. Indeed, it was suggested that changes to empower the 'customer' (that is, the patients) might have swung too far in the favour of the patient, to the detriment of effective general healthcare practice.

5. Since stress management interventions are likely to take time to implement, the introduction of a counselling service or employee assistance programmes should be made available to GPs who might become victims and casualties of exposure to stress at work. Some authorities have already provided counselling services to GPs. However, it would probably be useful to encourage GPs to use these services by sending a clear message that endorses the view that stress is an acceptable and important topic for action. It is necessary to acknowledge that problems are likely to exist but they can be dealt with in a positive and pro-active manner.

The nature of stress among doctors

As we have stated, the stress-management process must begin by first identifying the sources of stress, and then deciding on the course of action open. The tripartite model of stress management, described at the start of this chapter suggests we can try to do one or more of the following:

- eliminate or minimize the problem
- find ways to help doctors and medical staff to respond in more appropriate (that is, less damaging) ways to a source of stress that cannot be avoided

- help the doctor and staff who are already suffering from stress.

Thus, in the final part of this chapter we review some the studies that have investigated stress among doctors in order to prompt the stress-management thought processes.

Although sources of stress vary among doctors, the research evidence all points to the damaging nature of mismanaged stress. Doctors display signs of stress to a greater degree than normative groups in terms of:

- suicide rate – in young doctors (Richings et al. 1986); among senior doctors suicide rates are two to three times higher than in the general population (Beecham 2000); among women NHS doctors in the UK suicide rates are twice that of the general female population (Dobson 2001)
- drug or alcohol dependency – (Murray 1976, Allibone et al. 1981, Brooke et al. 1991)
- psychiatric disorders – anxiety and depression (Scheiber 1987, Caplan 1994, Beecham 2000)
- marital difficulties – (Scheiber 1987).

Whilst some studies suggest that doctors' physical health is better than for comparative groups (Allibone et al. 1981, British Medical Association 1993), the negative consequences of stress appear to spill over and can have an adverse impact on job performance, the well-being of doctors and patient care.

A review of the literature indicates that, while certain themes are evident, it is not possible to neatly generalize about stress among doctors, because sources of stress vary with type of medical practice and specialty. Nevertheless, in the next two sections we present some of the studies and findings on stress among hospital-based medical practitioners and doctors working in general and family practice.

Stress and hospital doctors

Studies of physicians have revealed job-related tension and reports of problems with patients, low levels of quality care and low job satisfaction. High workload, the need to work long hours, time pressures and inadequate free time emerge as key sources of strain in medical practice (Ford & Wentz 1986, Burke & Richardson 1990). In addition, the threat of malpractice suits, loss of autonomy, stricter regulations, disruptive events and professional development were also described as the antecedents of stress in medical settings in the USA (Richardson & Burke 1991). The pressure of working in a turbulent commercial, medical environment and the need to meet the demands imposed by change is ever present. Often the source of pressure appears to be more related to managerial skills (e.g. coping with patients' demands) than technical skills or related to other doctors in the work place. Nevertheless, the high clinical workload and stress at work was found to be a predictor of burnout among consultant doctors in Scotland (Deary et al. 1996).

Swanson and Power (1996) conducted a comparative study of consultant doctors (n = 449) and GPs (n = 547) in Scotland. It was carried out during a time of controversial change within primary and secondary care sectors of the UK NHS. Within the consultant group a total of fifty types of medical specialty were identified and categorized into the following groups:

- psychiatry (n = 72)
- anaesthetics (n = 51)
- radiology (n = 40)
- laboratory specialties (n = 35)
- managerial/public health (n = 45)
- general medical and surgical (n = 194).

No significant differences were found between these groups for levels of stress or job satisfaction. Simpson and Grant (1991) also noted this effect in their study conducted in the USA – that is, no significant differences in types of job stressors by medical specialty were noted. Whilst Swanson and Power did not find any differences in reported stress between the medical specialties among consultants, certain gender and age differences were noted.

In general practice and consultant specialties the male doctors worked longer hours and had heavier on-call commitments than their female colleagues (excluding female doctors who worked part-time).

This study used the Occupational Stress Indicator to measure stress levels and observed:

- Male doctors reported more stress intrinsic to the job and the job role than their female colleagues
- Consultant doctors reported the highest levels of stress associated with relationships with other people, career and achievement and the organizational structure and climate
- Relationships with colleagues at work and personal career development issues were key stressor and a source of job dissatisfaction for female consultants
- Younger doctors reported the highest levels of stress associated with the home–work interface. Other studies confirm this finding, but also observe that doctors in the youngest and the oldest age bands report the highest levels of home–work interface stress (Cooper et al. 1989; Wingfield and Anstey, 1991).

Ramirez et al. (1996) studied groups of gastroenterologists, surgeons, radiologists and oncologists, and found that the surgeons experienced the highest levels of both stress and job satisfaction, while the radiologists experienced the lowest levels. It was suggested that the radiologists, by the nature of their role as a clinical support service, receive less positive feedback from patients and relatives, and have less control over their work patterns. Anaesthetists are in a similar category and studies have found that their strongest source of stress is also this lack of control over working patterns, in addition to the sources of pressure faced by other doctors, such as, the pace of new developments, the stress of increased patient expectations and fear of litigation.

The work of anaesthetists has been examined for potential sources of stress since it involves considerable periods of monitoring, interspersed with periods of high demands on both physical and cognitive skills (Cooper et al. 1999). A study by Branton and Oborne 1979 observed that anaesthetists reported high levels of stress and fatigue at the end of a working day, but the evidence that they are more stressed than other medical practitioners is equivocal. Payne and Rick (1986) found that their stress levels were similar to surgeons, but they reported shorter periods of intense stress. The study of 564 anaesthetists by Cooper et al. (1999), found the stress of maintaining standards of patient care and communication within the hospital were rated as the greatest sources of pressure and had negative effects on job satisfaction and well-being. Likewise, research in the USA has suggested that some medical specialties, for example, anaesthetics and general family practice, are intrinsically more stressful than others, resulting in greater physician impairment (Talbott 1987). Overall, several studies suggest that anaesthetists are exposed to the same stressors as other medical practitioners, namely fear of litigation, the death of a patient, being audited, the pace of new developments in medicine and increased patient expectations; however, one specific source of stress is the lack of control over work patterns (McNamee et al. 1987, Dickson 1996, Seeley 1996).

Overall, the picture emerging is one of high stress, but often one of high satisfaction. Doctors appear to gain positive satisfaction from the intrinsic features of their work: exercising technical skills; mastering difficult problems; and the experience of responsibility, freedom and variety at work. It is suggested that such job satisfaction protects the medical practitioners' mental health against job stress (Lin et al. 1979, Cartwright & Anderson 1981, Rankin et al. 1987, Cooper et al. 1989, Clark et al. 1994, Ramirez et al. 1996, Swanson & Power 1996).

It is important to acknowledge the dynamic nature of stress and accept that stress and strain will vary according to career and life stage events. The sources of pressure that are evident in early stages of the career of a hospital doctor will differ from those reported by an experienced and mature, medical practitioner. Studies have shown that extended working hours and night working have long been the norm among junior house doctors, and are factors in the observed stress problems and poor mental health among this group (Spurgeon & Harrington 1989). The survey of junior house officers reported by Firth-Cozens and Morrison (1987) noted the following key sources of stress:

- dealing with death and dying
- relationships with senior doctors
- making mistakes
- being overworked
- relationships with ward staff
- lack of skills
- dealing with patients' relatives
- career decisions.

When asked how they dealt with these situations, they replied that they:

1. tackled the situation (29%)
2. asked for help (28% – most likely to be a strategy used by women rather than male doctors)
3. rationalized the event (13%)
4. failed to cope (12%)
5. dismissed the event (6%).

The most enjoyable aspect of the job for this group was 'feeling useful and interacting with patients'; least enjoyable was being overworked and having to do trivial tasks.

In the USA, research findings suggest (Reuben 1985) that approximately 33% of new doctors are depressed compared to 15% (using the same instrument) in community samples. Reuben reported that this percentage drops over subsequent years presumably as doctors become more experienced and confidant, and working hours are reduced. However, the need to acknowledge medical specialization was also highlighted by Reuben in this study since it was observed that levels of depression remained high among ICU second-year postgraduates. Thirty-seven percent of second-year ICU doctors had high levels of depression compared with 22% overall in the community.

Stress and GPs and family doctors

Considerable research evidence documents the strains and pressures associated with working in general practice (Cooper et al. 1989, Sutherland & Cooper 1992, 1993, Rout & Rout 1994, Chambers et al. 1996, Rout & Rout 1997, 2000, Sibbald et al. 2000). GPs report stress in many aspects of their working lives and the issues of concern are not only clinical. Pressures can be financial, legal, political and social. For example, one GP reported spending a considerable amount of time with the police because of suspected prescription forgeries and attempted thefts from the surgery (Sutherland & Cooper 1992). There is a general feeling that the profession is no longer in control of the things that impact upon their performance effectiveness and that non-medical considerations are assuming too much importance in the work role of the GP and family doctor. Research evidence also indicates that job dissatisfaction is consistently observed as an outcome of exposure to mismanaged stress. Since job satisfaction may be an important determinant of job performance (Grol et al. 1985) and physician retention and turnover (Lichenstein 1998), an understanding of the nature of stress among doctors is an important precursor in the effective management of stress.

The 'stress' picture that emerges describes the unpredictability of visiting patients; the apprehensions associated with caring for a wide diversity of people with different problems; having to make life or death instant decisions; occupational hazards, such as exposure to disease or infection; and the fear of violence towards GPs on call. It is clear that doctors face constant exposure to stress. In the UK, stress audits were conducted regularly among GPs during the 1990s, a period of considerable upheaval and change in the NHS. Table 2.2 shows the top fourteen sources of stress and the rank order in each, for surveys conducted in 1987, 1990 and 1998 respectively.

The overall picture from these three audits is one of decline in GP satisfaction from 1987 to 1990, followed by a partial recovery from 1990 to 1998 (Sibbald et al. 2000).

Table 2.2   GP stressors in 1987, 1990 and 1998

| | Rank order of items | | |
| | --- | --- | --- |
Item	1987 (n = 1817)	1990 (n = 917)	1998 (n = 999)
Dealing with problem patients	3	4	1
Worrying about patient complaints	5	8	2
Dividing time between work and family	8	5	3
Unrealistically high expectation of others	6	7	4
Disturbance of home/family life by GP work	4	3	5
Interruptions by emergency calls during surgery	1	2	6
Twenty-four hour responsibility for patients' lives	7	6	7
Finding a locum	11	13	8
Adverse publicity in the media	12	9	9
Arranging hospital admissions	9	10	10
Dealing with the terminally ill and their relatives	10	11	11
Night visits	2	1	12
Working environment, e.g. surgery set-up	14	12	13
Fear of assault during visits	13	14	14

Cited by Sibbald et al. (2000)

The NHS reforms of 1990/91 gave GPs greater managerial control and, of course, greater accountability. Not all GPs welcomed these changes (Leese & Bosanquet 1996) and job satisfaction levels deteriorated. Indeed, Sibbald et al. have suggested that clinical autonomy is a more important determinant of job satisfaction than managerial autonomy among medical professionals. Clearly, Table 2.2 indicates that dealing with problem patients and worrying about patient complaints have become prominent sources of stress for doctors, whilst the issue of 'night visits' appears to be less stressful. This may be attributable to the introduction of GP cooperatives for managing out-of-hours calls. Interruptions by emergency calls during surgery and disturbance to home and family life remain significant sources of stress and job dissatisfaction amongst

GPs. Family–job conflicts and disruption to social life continued to be key sources of strain well into the 1990s (Chambers et al. 1996). The comparative study of British GPs and Canadian family physicians also noted that time pressures, the demands on work and family life, and coping with difficult patients were significant sources of stress (Rout & Rout 1997). Likewise, Rout and Rout (2000) also observed that job satisfaction among GPs is still influenced by time pressure and interruptions, the working environment and communication, and career/goal achievement.

Since the 1990/1991 NHS reforms, some sources of stress have been removed or minimized, but the overall effect is perceived as a negative experience. The imposition of the 1990 GP contract by government was viewed as an attack on the independent contractor status and professional autonomy of GPs (Calnan & Williams 1995, Lewis 1997). Doctors were cynical and suspicious about the government's motives for change and believed that health improvement goals were secondary to financial constraints (Myerson 1993, Calnan & Williams 1995). In response to the increased workload levels and administrative demands (Hannay 1992, Leese & Bosanquet 1996) many practices have been forced to recruit more nurses, psychological counsellors, business administrators and other ancillary staff to help carry out some of the extra work associated with the reforms, particularly in relation to health promotion and disease prevention. Changes to levels of remuneration and method of payment have had varying effects on the levels of satisfaction and stress among doctors in general practice. Thus, doctors became fund holders, with the concomitant accountability and the role of resource allocation. This included responsibility for 'rationing' with a consequent pressure to move from a personal to a public ethos of doctoring (Royal College of General Practitioners 1996).

In addition, changes in the nature of the relationship between doctor and patient have also been identified as a cause of strain and pressure. The rise of consumerism within society has challenged the status of the medical practitioner since the patient has become a consumer, and the doctor is perceived as a service provider. Doctors now perceive that the patient has become more demanding, more discerning and less respectful of medical professionals (Calnan & Williams 1995). They feel the strain of worry about patients' complaints, the need to meet unrealistically high expectations, and adverse publicity in the media. Like many other professional groups, hospital doctors and GPs also face the prospect of clinical audit and appraisal. Whilst the purpose of this is to detect any problems of poor performance at an early stage and the protection of patients, the monitoring process is potentially a stressful experience. In the UK, the implementation of the working time directive, clinical governance, peer review and continuing professional development will decrease clinical time and increase stress levels. Thus, the challenge is to find ways of managing the stress that is intrinsic to the job of the medical professional.

An ability to accurately perceive demands and expectations is an important part of a stress-management programme. Since 'the patient' has been identified as a key source of stress for the doctor, in the final part of this chapter we consider some patients' views of doctors and medicine.

What does your patient think of you? Understanding patients' attitudes to doctors and medicine

Much has been written about doctor–patient relationships and the stress associated with difficult and demanding patients, patients who do not obey instructions, and the problems of dealing with the patients' relatives. In this section we consider the limited studies of patients' attitudes to doctors and medicine. We suggest that this should be considered an integral part of health psychology, since it attempts to provide an explanation of how people make use of medical services, and is relevant to the understanding of the nature of stress among doctors.

Doctors are a highly visible group and are used to the fact that most people have strong opinions and stereotypes concerning them and their profession (Conroy et al. 2002). The profession also receives considerable attention by the media, especially when the relationship between patient and doctor deteriorates or goes wrong. Praise and thanks are rarely highlighted or published, but dissatisfaction with diagnosis or treatment often is the subject of public attention and scrutiny. Likewise, studies of 'what the patient thinks' and patient satisfaction with medical services only receive media attention if a brickbat can be aimed at the medical profession. Therefore, it is useful to consider the research findings reported by Conroy et al. (2002), since they found that many perceptions about doctors varied according to whether the individual was asked to reflect on 'doctors in general', 'my family doctor' or 'my clinic (antenatal) doctor'. When the context changed from doctors in general to 'my family doctor' a number of positive changes in attitudes emerged. In this study, restricted to a sample of women, patients were much more likely to express confidence in the competence and effectiveness of their own doctor than in doctors in general. For example:

- Only 39% of the women agreed that 'all doctors are good doctors', compared to 85% of women in respect to their own family doctor, and nearly 97% expressing agreement about their clinic doctor.
- Only 45% agreed with the statement, 'I have absolute faith and confidence in all doctors', compared to 72% and 84% expressing agreement with this statement in respect to their family doctor and their clinic doctor respectively.
- Only 7.3% and 6.5% agreed with the statement, 'the doctor does too many unnecessary tests and investigations' with respect to their family doctor and their clinic doctor respectively, compared to nearly half of the group expressing agreement with this sentiment about doctors in general.

- Agreement with the statement, 'doctors blame their patients if their treatment doesn't work' did not vary significantly as a function of context: 12% agreed in respect to doctors in general, 11% in respect to the family doctor and 9% in respect to their clinic doctor.
- Only 9% of respondents agreed that they did not like doctors in general, compared to 16% who expressed this sentiment about their family doctor and nearly 4% who did not like their clinic doctor (Conroy et al. 2002).

As Conroy et al. explain, mothers attending antenatal clinics have quite a number of recent experiences of medicine and doctors in common, and do not consider themselves to be ill, nor are they. GP attendees, in contrast, generally have a specific health problem that may or may not be alleviated by a visit to their doctor. Nevertheless, this study serves as a useful reminder about the interpretation of studies that seek to find out and understand patients' perceptions about doctors and medicine. Clearly context plays a key role and explains the reason for the lack of unequivocal findings in such surveys. Likewise, McGee (1998) found that patient surveys consistently report high levels of satisfaction with particular episodes of care, compared to attitudes to care in general.

Whilst the premise of these authors is that attitudes are an important determinant of behaviour and surveys are potentially useful in understanding how patients will make use of medical services, quite clearly, care is needed in the construction, implementation and use of the findings arising from such surveys. At best, they can guide the doctor in providing care and medical services to their patients, at worst, they create stress for doctors, impoverish the relationship between doctor and patient, and provide fuel for the media to reinforce the negative perceptions of doctors and medicine held by the public.

The perceived expertise of the doctor also appears to be an influencing factor in the reported attitude of the patient to medicine and their doctor. Patients present to doctors with a variety of stress-related health problems.

Increasingly, many of these are psychosocial and psychological disorders. Further, it is suggested that psychiatric and psychological problems presenting in general practice consultations are frequently not recognized (Freeling et al. 1985, Ormel et al. 1989, Goldberg & Huxley 1992). Also, GPs are not universally perceived as appropriate providers of care in these circumstances. Research evidence suggests that there are a number of potential barriers to the presentation of psychiatric disorders, including patient embarrassment and concerns about doctors' lack of training and their reactions to such presentations (Priest et al. 1996). More recently, Bower et al. (1999) have conducted research into patients' perceptions of the role of the GP in the management of emotional problems. The Physician Belief Scale was modified for use by patients and was called the Patient Perceptions Scale (PPS). A 16-item questionnaire was designed to measure the following factors:

- Perceptions of the doctor's role.
- What patients want and do not want in relation to emotional care.
- Doctors' reactions to patients with emotional problems.

In this investigation the word 'psychosocial' problem was changed to 'emotional' problem to avoid jargon. Fifteen of the items formed fours factors namely:

1. Patients' perceptions of the GPs' orientation to the management of emotional problems:
   a. the GP can treat emotional problems
   b. the GP always looks for physical problems before asking about emotional ones
   c. the GP only tries to deal with physical problems
   d. when the doctor sees patients, the doctor looks for emotional problems as well as physical problems.
2. Patients' preferences concerning the GPs' role in the management of emotional problems:
   a. I want to ask the doctor about emotional problems
   b. it is the business of the GP to ask his patients about any emotional problems

    c. the stresses of everyday life can make us ill

    d. people often go to the GP with aches and pains when the real problem is emotional.

3. Perceived workload implications of the management of emotional problems:

    a. if the GP treats emotional problems, the doctor will have too much work on his hands

    b. if the GP tries to help with emotional problems, people might come to rely on the doctor too much

    c. the GP is too pressed for time to investigate emotional problems regularly.

4. Perceived GP reaction to the management of emotional problems:

    a. the GP can only help with emotional problems if the doctor had to sort out similar problems for him/herself

    b. if the GP asked about emotional problems I would not go to see the doctor

    c. if the GP deals with patients' emotional problems, the doctor is likely to become upset

    d. the GP can only deal with emotional problems if the doctor does not have such problems him/herself.

Note: two versions of this scale were constructed depending on the gender of the participating GP (Bower et al. 1999). We have used the word 'doctor', and 'him' and 'herself' in the above item descriptions.

The results of this survey of 1511 patients and 43 GPs indicated that female patients reported preferences for, and positive perceptions of, the GPs' orientation to emotional issues. They were also less likely to report that the GPs' emotional reactions were an important barrier to care. Patients with high GHQ scores (the General Health Questionnaire is a psychiatric screening measure – high scores denotes psychiatric cases) were more likely to prefer their GPs to have a role in emotional care, which strengthens the GPs' potential role (Bower et al. 1999). Also, elderly patients had a more positive attitude to the GPs' emotional role than the younger respondents in this survey.

Stress among doctors – conclusion

The need to see more and more patients, meet high administrative demands and deal with ever increasing non-clinical matters continues without signs of abatement. Doctors are increasingly dissatisfied with the amount of time they can spend with patients. A recent survey by the Commonwealth Fund (2000) found that three-quarters of doctors in the five countries studied believed that spending more time with patients is a highly effective way to improve patient care. Evidence indicates that longer consultations are of a higher quality (Howie et al. 1999) and are wanted by patients. Yet, according to Smith (2000), 62% of doctors in the UK, 43% in the USA, 42% in Canada, 38% in Australia, and 32% in the Commonwealth Fund study, reported that not having enough time with patients is a major problem. The NHS system in the UK, the government sponsored, single payer system in Canada, the mandatory insurance systems in Continental Europe and Japan, and the managed care systems in the USA, all appear to create patient overload problems for doctors and their staff. Doctors are finding these systems exhausting – many are leaving medical practice. Negative media attention has also led to problems with the recruitment of new doctors, particularly in the UK, and many of those doctors who remain are disillusioned. As one single, female consultant surgeon reflected in Dumelow's study (2000):

I would not start my medical career again. It's taken too much out of me. You don't have a life outside medicine, where other priorities seem not to weigh up. There is no pot of gold at the end of the rainbow. There are other ways of living too.

The need to redesign health care to overcome this problem is evident, but the process is too slow. Therefore, whilst acknowledging the key issue of work overload, it is also necessary to use a stress diagnosis process to understand individual vulnerability or risk and to identify the other sources of strain and pressure that exist in medical practice. An audit or analysis guides the doctor to ways of self-managing stress, or to remove or minimize the risks associated with exposure to stress. We believe that a strategy that identifies stress and attempts to prevent potential problems is more effective and efficient than trying to cure victims of exposure to stress. It is about optimizing the performance, health and work–life balance of doctors exposed to change and the demands of society in the 21st century.

part TWO

Managing stress in your work environment

The next two chapters address the topics of working practices and the actual work environment of the doctor. The first is a recommendation to improve your time-management behaviour in the workplace and the second addresses the actual working conditions and physical workplace of the doctor.

A state of stress might exist because we have too much to do in the time available and often we exacerbate this situation because we do not manage our time as effectively as we might. Most people become prickly with irritation when it is suggested that their stress might be the result of failure to manage their time or the work environment effectively. It is an unpalatable truth that most of us would rather deny. Also, many doctors initially complain that time management, as a strategy, is not likely to be a useful stress-management option for them because they do not have discretionary time. Nevertheless, our personal experience of running time-management courses for doctors has encouraged us to include this as a potentially useful stress-management strategy. Following attendance on a time-management course, many doctors and their practice staff and administrative support personnel have subsequently admitted that taking time out to assess how they really used their time had been a revelation and the spur to motivate change. Also, the tips and time-management tricks helped as part of a stress-coping strategy. However, we believe it is important to emphasize that this type of approach to the management of stress is not a miracle cure – rather it should be viewed as a means of easing the strain from a pressure cooker. By such techniques the pressure cooker will remain safe while exposed to heat. Only by removing the heat can it ever be completely safe from explosion, harm and complete destruction. This, we feel is an appropriate analogy for doctors in their current work situation. It is not possible to remove the heat, but the pressure can be controlled without experiencing serious and dramatic short-term or permanent harm.

We have suggested that the improved time-management behaviour can potentially lessen the impact of stressors for doctors. However, we also acknowledge that doctors and their staff and associates, like many other professionals, often work in conditions that exacerbate stress without realizing the negative effect that the environment is having on performance effectiveness and well-being. For this reason we offer some guidance in Chapter four on creating an effective work environment.

Time management

Evaluation research into the effectiveness of time management as a stress-management option is limited, but evidence exists to indicate that engaging in time-management behaviour has a positive impact on mental health, and this may be due to enhanced feelings of control (Lang 1992, Macan 1994, Jex & Elecqua 1999). For example, Lang (1992) found that time-management coping behaviours were associated with lower levels of depression, anxiety and physical symptoms. Macan (1994) found that engaging in effective time-management behaviour was associated with lower levels of job tension, somatic tension and higher levels of job satisfaction. Before we describe the elements of a time-management system, the issues of workload, long hours of working and burnout among doctors are discussed in the next two sections.

Workload and long hours of working as sources of stress

The reorganization of work-time arrangements has been a key feature of economic structuring for many professionals working in healthcare. For many doctors this has created a work overload condition and the need to work long hours. A review of the long work-hours literature has found a relationship between prolonged work hours and employee mental and physical ill health (Sparks et al. 1997, 2001). It is arguable that the relation between work hours and ill health is mediated by stress, and long hours act both directly and indirectly as a stressor. The direct impact is to increase the demands on the doctor who attempts to maintain performance levels in the face of increasing fatigue, and indirectly by increasing the time that the doctor is exposed to other sources of workplace stress. A high level of stress has long been acknowledged as a contributory factor in the development of certain types of psychiatric problems, heart disease, musculoskeletal problems and symptoms associated with gastrointestinal problems. The last of these problems tends to be exacerbated by night-shift working, disruption to eating habits and subsequent digestive problems.

Stress as time pressure, having too much work to do, and the need to work long hours features high on the list of key sources of strain for doctors working in hospital environments and in general practice (Ford & Wentz 1986, Firth-Cozens 1987, Reese & Cooper 1992, Kirkcaldy et al. 1997, Beecham 2000). In a qualitative survey of hospital consultants in the UK (Dumelow 2000) one doctor reflected:

> *The long hours are very damaging; you tend to fall into a routine of work, eat, sleep, and you become alienated. The rewards to an individual can be tremendous but at great personal sacrifice in terms of life outside medicine (Single, male, childless, diagnostics consultant) (cited Dumelow 2000).*

The long duty hours of trainee doctors have also received attention, with studies reporting both health and performance impairments (Spurgeon & Harrington 1989, Scott 1992, Firth-Cozens 1993). Leonard et al. (1998) assessed the effects of a 32-hour on-call shift on pre-registration house doctors in Ireland and found that the lack of sleep adversely affected psychological well-being and the ability of the junior doctors to carry out simple tasks on alertness and concentration. Research in other workers suggests that loss of sleep rather than long hours of work is the problem, causing decrements in mood and performance (Arnetz et al. 1990, Firth-Cozens 1993). Also, the quality of sleep is important and studies indicate that this is inferior in those on call, expecting to be woken, who show greater sleepiness the following day (Torsvall & Akerstedt 1988). A national study of consultants in accident and emergency medicine in the UK found that being overstretched, the effect of hours and stress on family life, and lack of recognition were strong predictors of mental health 'caseness'. In this study, 154 respondents (44.4%) had scores over the threshold for distress (a definition of 'caseness'). This was much higher than in other studies of doctors. The researchers found that long working hours were directly linked to self-reported, poor mental well-being (Burbeck et al. 2001). It is clear, long periods of on call and broken sleep are detrimental to both doctor and patient. Whilst certain central UK directives have attempted to reduce working hours for doctors, particularly junior doctors, the situation is not resolved. Stress levels remain high and satisfaction with shift systems in the UK is far from positive (Baldwin et al. 1997). A review of research into work-related stress by the British Medical Association found that NHS consultants work on average 50 plus hours a week for the NHS, with one in three routinely working more than 60 hours. Many senior doctors are struggling to maintain high-quality services to patients in the face of excessive workload. The stress is serious enough to affect their health and impair their ability to provide high-quality care to patients, with nearly half of GPs showing symptoms of distress (Beecham 2000).

Time management for doctors

Whilst the issue of long hours of working for doctors needs to be addressed through government, legislation and working-time directives, we acknowledge that a perfect solution to this problem is unlikely. In any event, strategic change is likely to be a slow process and an imperfect resolution. Consequently, we believe that doctors will continue to work long hours and be exposed to heavy workloads in the foreseeable future. Employer demands, patient expectations, economic restructuring, the need to keep abreast of medical and technological developments, and an inability to fill posts, will all add to the workload demands on the doctor.

Therefore, in this chapter we recommend the use of time-management strategies as an option for the management of work overload stress and as an adaptive stress coping mechanism. Further, it is suggested by Jex and Bliese (1999) that the provision of training in self-efficacy, and individuals with a strong self-efficacy (defined as an individual's beliefs regarding the likelihood that a particular course of action or behaviour can be carried out) report less physical and psychological strain with long work hours and work overload compared to those with lower self-efficacy. Therefore, where long hours are unavoidable, training in self-efficacy and time management will help an individual to gain control over time and a sense of personal mastery of a potentially stressful situation.

Having more work to do than a person can accomplish in the time available is described as 'quantitative overload' or role overload. As business strives to become more effective by de-manning, many of us find ourselves doing more and more, with restricted resources – and this is the plight of the medical practitioner. In addition to role overload, the pressures of fulfilling multiple roles generate demands on our time and so the doctor will be required to meet the demands of the job, a family and social life. This type of overload, and 'time-conflict', has long been recognized as a cause of psychological and physical strain (Kahn et al. 1964). Time-management interventions are widely recommended for increasing personal productivity and may be helpful in preventing overload strain. Evaluation studies of time management have indicated that it can help to reduce tension and strain in the form of anxiety. Individuals who invest in time management report feeling more in control of their lives. They believe that they achieve more because they spend less time trying to catch up on things and in fire fighting! Feeling overwhelmed by work and controlled by the strains and the pressures of medical practice can lead to burnout. This is discussed in the next section.

Identifying job burnout

Theoretically it is assumed that burnout results from the emotional demands of interacting with other people (Maslach 1993). Pines and Aronson (1988) define burnout as a state of physical, emotional and mental exhaustion caused by long-term involvement in situations that are emotionally demanding. These are described as follows:

- Physical exhaustion – characterized by low energy, chronic fatigue and weakness.
- Emotional exhaustion – this involves primarily feelings of helplessness, hopelessness and entrapment.
- Mental exhaustion – characterized by the development of negative attitudes towards one's self, work and life itself.

Therefore, burnout is characterized by emotional exhaustion, depersonalization and feelings of reduced personal accomplishment. Burnout can be identified as:

1. Feeling physically and emotionally weary or exhausted – 'TATT' syndrome, that is feeling 'tired all the time'. This means consistently feeling exhausted at the end of the day, low energy levels and weakness; having trouble falling asleep because you cannot 'switch-off'.
2. Feeling overwhelmed – for example, feeling that you have too much responsibility; constantly working under pressure.
3. Feeling unhappy – for example, not having enough time to do the things that you normally enjoyed.
4. Feeling worthless or hopeless – for example, not having enough time to complete your work effectively.
5. Feeling trapped – for example, feeling that you cannot take 'it' anymore; not seeing any way out.
6. Feeling disillusioned and resentful towards other people – for example, feeling that patients, family or friends (and/or people in general) expect too much of you; feeling a lack of compassion, also known as 'empathy fatigue'.
7. Feeling depressed.
8. Feeling rejected – for example, not having people to assist and support you.

9. Feeling anxious – for example, realizing that you are becoming forgetful or indecisive.
10. Feeling troubled without specific cause.
11. Feeling demoralized – for example, negative attitudes towards self, work and life itself; loss of motivation; just going through the motions, not completely attuned to patients' physical or emotional needs.
12. Feeling negative about oneself and other people – for example, wanting to distance yourself from other people

How often did you experience any of the above symptoms of burnout in the past 3 months? Compare these responses to the times you are able to report that you went to work and:

1. felt happy
2. had a good day
3. felt energetic
4. felt optimistic.

Naturally the issue of 'time-frame' is problematic (Enzmann et al. 1998) and it differs for us all. Thus, the suggestion to reflect back over the past 3 months may not be relevant for your personal circumstances. Also the symptoms and responses described above, individually, are expected and a normal reaction to difficult and distressful events in the life and work of the medical professional. Thus, this list can be used only as a guide to prompt personal reflection and to act as an alert when a change occurs in your behaviour that significantly affects your ability to cope. When several of these symptoms occur simultaneously, over a period of time, it may signal the early stages of a burnout condition. Since many of the physical and emotional symptoms of stress and burnout are denied by the Type A coronary-prone doctor, it is important that particular attention is paid to this potentially deleterious condition. Therefore, it is suggested that Type A doctors encourage a colleague or spouse/partner to speak out if they observe symptoms of potential burnout that the individual doctor is unaware of personally or would rather try to ignore.

The problem of burnout among doctors is acknowledged as a serious problem. In addition to the personal costs associated with physical and psychological ill health, according to Crane (1998), insurers have recognized that burned-out physicians are more likely to make mistakes than their 'more mellow colleagues', and so become, a 'lawsuit waiting to happen'. Learning to cope with burnout is, therefore, identified as a liability-prevention strategy, and in the USA insurance carriers are sponsoring stress-reduction seminars (Crane 1998). Also, the cost of finding and recruiting a replacement for a burned-out or impaired doctor can be immense.

Passineau (cited in Crane 1998) states that burnout and malpractice creates a cycle of continuing stress and business losses. Once a malpractice claim is filed against a physician, the chance of that doctor being involved in a subsequent incident that will result in another lawsuit increases significantly during the following year.

The issue of stress-management strategies is dealt with in the final chapter of this book. However, it is appropriate at this point to identify certain steps to avoid burnout:

1. Monitor and control your hours of working – maintain a good work–life balance. If your workload is to blame for your burnout and you cannot meet your daily patient quota or the on-call schedule, you will need to try and renegotiate your workload. Your employer has a duty of care to ensure that you do not become damaged physically or psychologically as a result of work overload and burnout, and should respond appropriately to avoid the cost of burnout to the doctor, the medical system and the patients. Remember that, in addition to patient care, you need to budget time for professional and personal development, including update reading AND a social life outside of medical practice. The next section on time management and the recommended use of a time log will help you to recognize when certain activities become counterproductive due to fatigue.

2. Emphasize your people skills – be aware that a lack of empathy is a sign of burnout. Make sure that you are really listening to your patients; make eye contact; do not write or use the computer while the patient is talking (Passineau, cited in Crane 1998).

3. Realize that you are not perfect – Bartlett (cited in Murray 2000) suggests that people who choose a career as demanding as medicine are, by nature, compulsive and perfectionist. Medical training feeds these tendencies and so by the time the doctor is in private practice, the notion that you can do it all often extends to family as well as practice. This is an unrealistic and unhealthy assumption that can result in burnout. Bartlett suggests that doctors must strive for excellence rather than perfection.

4. Use the support of colleagues and family – ensure that you maintain strong social support networks at home and at work; consult with colleagues over difficult cases; communicate your hopes and fears, openly with a spouse, partner or close friend; do not bottle-up your emotions. Make use of professional counselling services.

5. Do not let petty annoyances sap your energy – if every perceived outrage sends you into an emotional spin, you are more likely to become a casualty of burnout. Try not to become enraged if someone uses your parking space or the hospital canteen runs short of the meal you would have chosen. Allow the system to deal with your complaint, or as Cejka (1999) suggests, you should learn to pick your battles and shrug off the rest – life is too short to be in a constant state of stress.

6. Monitor your use of alcohol and drugs – under extreme stress we are more likely to resort to maladaptive coping strategies and so might become vulnerable to addiction.

7. If you are bored, do something to recharge your interest (Cejke 1999). Complaint of terminal ennui cannot be cured necessarily by a new job, because this will probably become routine eventually. If you are bored by the routine of day-to-day medicine try to challenge yourself, take a course to learn a new skill, or make the job more stimulating.

8. Incorporate regular physical activity into your life – as Cejka (1999) suggests, candidates for burnout tend to be seriously out of shape. The benefits of exercise as a stress-management strategy are well documented and you will feel better both physically and mentally if you take regular exercise (refer to final chapter for details on exercise as a stress-coping strategy).

In the next section we describe the elements of a time-management system and how it might be of practical use to the medical professional.

Elements of a time-management system

An old parable tells of a man who insists on using a leaky bucket to carry water. Each time he gets to his destination, the bucket is nearly empty. Finally, someone asks him why he won't take a few minutes to repair it, 'I can't,' the man snarls. 'I'm too busy carrying the water.' According to Murray (2000) many doctors can relate to this tale. For example, he suggests that doctors are guilty of overbooking and then leaving the office or surgery at 8 pm rather than 6 pm; they do not delegate when there is an opportunity; they agree to chair yet another committee rather than decline to become involved. For some, this style of behaviour (note, these are also classic patterns of behaviour for the Type A coronary-prone doctor) might lead to some cataclysmic event such as the break-up of a marriage, serious or even a fatal illness. However, Murray also believes that in the absence of a major life catastrophe many doctors respond by abusing drugs, alcohol or both. The need to acknowledge that it is possible to take control of the strains and pressures of working in medical practice is one of the first steps to successful stress management. Through the technique of time management we are able to gain control by understanding how time is managed, used and lost.

Macan et al. (1990) suggest that time-management behaviour can be broken down into three dimensions, namely:

1. Goal setting and prioritization – deciding what it is to be accomplished each day and what is important.
2. Mechanics of time management – activities such as making lists and preparing for work.
3. Preference for organization – have a methodical and systematic approach to work. Essentially, time-management behaviour is a form of active coping that may buffer the effects of multiple or conflicting job demands by enhancing doctors preparedness (Carver et al. 1989, Leiter 1991).

Typically, the control of time is achieved through the following six actions:

1. The development of goals
2. Planning
3. Prioritizing
4. The scheduling of time
5. Avoiding interruptions and distractions
6. Delegation.

It is suggested that effective time management will help you to:

1. develop a personal sense of time
2. think about and set realistic and achievable goals
3. analyze where, how and why you are spending your time at present
4. reduce time pressures
5. rid yourself of activities that waste time
6. delegate effectively
7. learn time-saving techniques in meetings, reading, travel, telephone calls and scheduling, etc.
8. use time more creatively
9. find time to relax and enjoy life
10. make time an ally instead of an enemy (Adair 1982).

Recognize the need to improve your time-management behaviour

Time management has many facets. However, the following brief questionnaire will provide the danger signals of poor time management. Answer 'Yes' or 'No' to the following questions.

- I feel constant pressure because I am always trying to catch up.
- I regularly miss deadlines.
- I regularly take work home.
- I feel overwhelmed by the demands on my time.
- I am indispensable.
- My schedule does not go according to plan because of constant interruptions.
- Life seems to go from crisis to crisis.
- I always have too much to do because I find it difficult to say no.
- I often put off doing things because I cannot face the task.
- Meetings always seem to overrun the scheduled time.
- It is more exciting doing several tasks at the same time.
- Colleagues are constantly chasing me for information or paperwork.
- I never seem to have enough time for rest.
- I feel guilty if I am not on the go all of the time.
- I frequently seem to be doing several things at a time.
- I am the only one who can do my job.
- Sometimes I find that I'm not listening to other people.
- My problems are caused by unrealistic deadlines.
- I am always rushing.
- I misplace items.
- There is never enough time to plan .... I am always 'fire fighting'.

If you answered 'yes' to at least six or seven of the above questions it is likely that some improvement in your time-management skills would help you to achieve a better work–life balance, and reduce strain and pressure at work and home.

Diagnosing time-management problems

We need to understand how we spend time in order to use it more effectively. Until we take some time to analyze where time goes we probably do not realize how much we waste time and/or fail to use it effectively and efficiently. The best way to achieve this is to keep a time log. However, many people feel that this just adds to their stress levels. Initially, you might prefer to assess the need for better time management by answering the following questions:

- What frustrates me about my job?
- What do I want from my job?
- What am I not getting from my job or way of life?
- What am I doing too much of/too little of?
- What are my priorities?
- What are my three greatest time wasters?
- How often do I lose time through interruptions?
- Am I satisfied with my job and my work–life balance?
- Where do I want to be 1 year/5 years from now?
- Did I achieve my objective today/this week/this month?

Honest answers to these questions may provide the motivation for taking part in a 'time-log' exercise.

Using a time log

A time log is a detailed record of how you currently spend your day. Since this can become an onerous and sometimes demoralizing task, it is important to design a log that is easily completed with minimum effort. Begin by producing a list of all the jobs that need to be done, all the activities that fill your day/week, including activities such as, journey times, talking with colleagues, telephone calls and work breaks. It is usual for people attending a time-management course to complete a log for a 7-day period, however, this will depend on the duration of your typical work cycle. A time log should identify the:

- amount of time spent in various activities
- purpose of the activity – did it contribute to your effectiveness as a doctor?
- necessity of the activity – did the task need to be done, done at that time, did YOU need to do it?

- other people involved in your daily activities – how they facilitate or inhibit your effectiveness
- outcomes – did you achieve your goal: were you successful, effective, satisfied and happy?

Analysis of the time log will reveal any discrepancies between reality and your work plan or goals for the day. It will highlight interruptions, failure to delegate, and the ways in which other people disrupted your schedule. Ultimately, it should be possible to use your time log to identify the source of disruptions and enable you to prioritize key activities. This type of time-log approach was used by the authors in the study of job stress, satisfaction and mental health among GPs after the introduction of new contracts (Sutherland & Cooper 1992). A small sub-group of GPs completed time-log diaries for a period of 2 weeks. Analysis of the logs indicated that GPs were not spending as much time on non-clinical work as they had perceived initially. It was felt that the new contract forced the GP to spend more time on non-clinical activities and was a key course of stress. Thus, the findings were an unexpected outcome for GPs, but not for the researchers. Typically, we have found that respondents will overestimate the amount of time spent on activities that are either disliked or imposed, but underestimate the time spent on preferred and enjoyable work tasks.

Appendix II provides an example of a simple time log as a guideline. Although the process seems laborious, it becomes easier with practice and can be a very worthwhile exercise in the stress-management process. You can also produce a checklist by dividing each day into 15-minute intervals; at the end of each hour you record what you were doing during that period of time. An activities list would be listed across the top of the sheet, thus forming a grid. However, this 'tick-list' might not provide the wealth of information needed to help formulate an action plan. It is suggested that you begin with a simple checklist and then move on to a more detailed version when you become more comfortable with the process of logging time.

When you have completed your time log, or after 3 or 4 days of entries, it is possible to examine the various activities, calculate the amount of time spent on each and rank these in importance to your effectiveness as a doctor. Table 3.1 below illustrates this summary process: list all of the activities, the time taken and the percentage of time spent in each activity. Then rank the activities by listing the most important as rank one, and so on. This type of analysis will identify if you are taking too long to complete relatively unimportant activities and/or how much discretionary time you actually have available. It also prevents us from remaining blinkered about the ways in which we actually use time.

Cejka (1999) suggests that doctors often have trouble when they attempt to produce a list of responsibilities in order of importance because they view everything as important. For example, a list might include, serving on a hospital committee, seeing patients, doing charts and ordering supplies, and typically the doctor finds it impossible to prioritize this list. However, Cejka maintains that the doctor does have three top priorities, the need to see patients, the need to do charts, and the need to prevent yourself from wearing out so that you can keep seeing patients and doing charts! As we have already mentioned, we are often sub-consciously guilty of engaging in faulty thinking because we tend to believe that disliked activities take longer than they do in reality, and the opposite is the case for enjoyable tasks of course. The use of a time log challenges such unrealistic assumptions. The final column of a time log is used to specify problems, make decisions about remedial actions and plan new goals.

Table 3.1 Summary of time-log activities

Your activity	Amount of time spent	% total time	Ranking	Problem/actions/goals

Action planning

The next step is to make an action plan to improve your time-management behaviour. By identifying the importance of each activity you can prepare a list that prioritizes your daily activities and sets a time budget for each. It is important to acknowledge that you do not need to be a slave to other people's schedules (Cejka 1999). Not every patient must be seen today and a good receptionist can respond to your instructions on which types of patients should receive priority. If you are absolutely certain that you need to deal personally with suppliers, computer salespeople and other non-patients, schedule meetings at your convenience, not theirs, and set strict time limits for each meeting. It helps to rate each activity: clearly some activities are essential and so would be graded 'A' ('must do'); however, close scrutiny might permit you to downgrade an activity to either 'B' ('should do'), or even a 'C' ('might do; do only in crisis'), or 'D' ('don't do'). You will probably need more than these four categories, for example, subgroups such as A1, A2, A3 etc. Your action plan must identify your priorities and clear goals.

Work smarter not harder!

An action plan for the day, week or month should identify your goals and objectives and describe how you plan to realize these aims. For example, plan to complete charts and records after each consultation is complete and within your scheduled workday. Some doctors try to maximize the number of patients they see by saving all chart writing until the last patient has left and then they sacrifice the evening by doing the charts after hours. As Cejka (1999) suggests, this is an invitation to burnout. In following certain time-management rules we can aim to work 'smarter' not harder. It is worth noting at this point that certain personality types, namely the Type A coronary-prone individual, tend to create stress because they constantly set unrealistic goals. We address this in detail in Chapter six when we examine the link between behaviour and stress. The following advice on goal setting is particularly important for Type As, but a useful stress-management strategy for everyone.

Set SMART goals – review progress

SMART means:

- Specific – clear, consistent, written
- Measurable
- Achievable – challenging and worthwhile
- Realistic – attainable and agreed by all parties involved (many doctors work to exhaustion because they do not set realistic life goals; thus the need to reevaluate lifestyle priorities is an important part of the goal-setting exercise)
- Time-bounded.

It should also be remembered that achievement of a goal, set for an individual or group of people, is more likely to be achieved if the individual, or members of the group actually take some part in this process by helping to specify and agree the target or goal. Research evidence indicates that under such conditions, higher targets are likely to be set and achieved if the process is 'participative' rather than as 'assigned' goals. At an agreed time it is necessary to review progress and assess the goal outcomes. If your objectives were not met, the reason for failure must be established. Limited success might be due to

- circumstances beyond your control – could these have been identified earlier?
- circumstances within your control – were warning signs ignored? Why did you fail to adjust the plan? Remember a plan is something from which to deviate if circumstances change, so stay flexible
- lack of motivation – identify the reasons for your difficulties
- inappropriate deadlines – lack of skill or resources to complete the task.

Make and use lists

Effective time management means having a written 'life plan'. The basic requirements of a time plan are to define what one has to do, how it should be done and when it should happen. Typically a life plan should describe your long- and short-term goals and include:

- a 3- or 5-year plan for your future
- your objectives for the forthcoming year
- a plan of activities for the next month, by week
- a daily to-do list – it is suggested that this is best done the evening before so that you can sleep on it. After sleep and a rest from work you might want to review the list and alter some of your priorities. The to-do list should be arranged or marked in some order of priority (considering both urgency and importance), and you should set a time limit for each activity. You might need to accept that you are guilty of procrastination if you find that you continually transfer an item from the list to the next days' activities. At the end of the day review the list and ask if things did not get done because there were simply too many items on the list, or because you were not ready to tackle the item. A task might have been avoided because you were unsure about what to do, you felt bored by it or the task seemed to be too difficult. By removing these barriers to your personal effectiveness you are more likely to complete a task and feel satisfied and happy with the outcome.

The most common reason for not achieving one's goals and objectives is due to 'interruptions'. In the next section we consider certain time wasters and suggest ways of controlling this problem.

Manage time-waster interruptions

The need to be accessible to patients will limit the usefulness of this option for doctors. However, the use of a time log will indicate if you are interrupted at other times.

- Too many interruptions – define and establish a quiet time when you can work undisturbed. Your time budget for the day will guide your actions. Decide what is the most important, your planned job or the interruption. Agree and establish an open-door policy and the rules. This does not mean that you are available to everyone for every minute of the day.
- Drop-in callers – establish the times you are prepared to accept callers. Ask for someone to screen callers, close your door and schedule breaks to meet or socialize with colleagues. Stand up to greet an unexpected caller and remain standing to avoid a lengthy interruption. If it looks as if more time will be needed for the discussion, suggest making an appointment for dealing with this unplanned activity at another time. It also helps to develop the habit of going to the other person's work area because you can leave when you want to. If you find it difficult to get rid of an unwanted visitor, arrange to be interrupted by someone else.
- Learn to say no more often – be honest, polite and sensitive. It does not mean that we are advising you to stop helping people. Effectiveness at work means knowing what not to do, because over-commitment will have an adverse effect on your performance and health. Your own success depends on learning to say no with tact and firmness. It usually helps to give a reason when saying no. Avoid being vague to ensure that the other person is not unclear about your intentions. This might lead to misunderstandings and future disappointment if they wrongly expect help.
- The telephone – this probably does rule the life of the doctor during the day and night, because there is a need to respond, irrespective of what else is happening! However, there are times when this is not the case and certain rules can ensure that the telephone does not waste your time. Be ruthless and decide whether you need to answer the call personally. Arrange for another person to screen and deal with your calls. Establish a time and place for accepting and making telephone

calls. Respect the other person you are calling by asking at the onset if they have time to speak and encourage this habit as part of your telephone interactions. Learn to terminate a call that is wasting time by being assertive. Close the call on an action point and be positive and constructive. Plan and decide what your objective is before making a call. It builds trust and confidence if you always call someone back when you say you will.

- Indecision is a time waster – gather information and give yourself a deadline; accept that you are human and that risk is part of the human condition. Mistakes in medical practice are 'the unthinkable', but acknowledge that none of us is 100% perfect 100% of the time.
- Lack of planning – ensure you have a daily to-do list. Make sure that you try to do the most important tasks when your energy levels are the highest. This, of course, is not a realistic suggestion for the doctor on call. However, it is possible to plan for the call out by ensuring that the routine, anticipated aspects of a call out are scheduled and dealt with in advance.
- Paper shuffling – only handle paperwork once. Every time you pick up a piece of paper, deal with it, file it, or throw it away!
- Procrastination – sometimes we waste time because we cannot face starting a big task that appears to be too daunting because we fear failure. These are known as 'elephant' tasks and it is useful to remember the advice on how to eat an elephant! That is, 'one bite at a time'. Plan and organize to break down that daunting job into manageable 'bites'. Make sure that you work on one 'bite' of this each day for a set period of time. Reward yourself at stages throughout the job. As Mark Twain said, 'If you have to eat frog, don't look at it too long. If you have to eat two frogs, eat the big one first.'
- Routine and low importance tasks, known as 'the ants' – it is easy to waste time on routine, or easy tasks, usually because they act as a displacement activity from

the urgent and import things that are more difficult to tackle. As Parkinson's second law states, 'We tend to devote time and energy to tasks in inverse relation to their importance.' Save such tasks and deal with lots of 'ants' in one session, in non-prime time, and when your energy levels are low. It is suggested that we are more likely to complete a series of tasks, in the faster time, if we begin by doing something easy – next do something nasty – and then follow this by doing something nice. Do not leave the nasty and difficult 'ants' all to the end.

- Inability to delegate – we waste our time by doing a task that could and should be done by someone else. Delegate when possible and do not do unnecessary tasks.
- Avoid having a cluttered work area – only have the items you are currently using in front of you (the management of the work environment is discussed further in the next chapter).
- Meetings can be a great time waster – this is the topic of the next section.

Managing meetings

Many of us find ourselves attending more and more meetings, and frequently complain about the amount of time wasted in meetings. As we move towards a more consultative work culture, where medical practitioners work in multidisciplinary teams, the need for meetings will remain paramount. However, there are ways of managing meetings to make them more effective and less likely to be a waste of your time. We suggest that you begin by producing a meeting analysis to decide if the meeting is actually necessary, and whether you need attend. Complete the pro-forma that follows, developed by John Adair (1982), for each meeting:

1. Purpose of the meeting. Briefly, write down the objectives and aims of the meeting. This will help you to decide if your personal input is necessary. If you only need to know what happened in the meeting then you could simply read the minutes at a later date and save time by not attending.

2. People in attendance. Meetings are often unproductive because too many members attend. A review helps you decide the necessary, minimal numbers in attendance. Also, we sometimes go to a meeting out of habit or because we fear a loss of power by not attending. People should be allowed to leave a meeting if their part is finished.

3. Frequency and average duration. The meeting analysis is used to help you and your group decide on the frequency of regular meetings. Many meetings are still held without an agenda and a timetable. People dread attending some meetings because they do not have a specified time budget and are unstructured. A detailed agenda with a given objective and timetable should be prepared for ALL meetings and circulated in advance. Meetings should always start and finish on time and keep to the agenda. If you delay the start of a meeting by waiting for latecomers you are likely to perpetuate this bad behaviour – so start without them!

4. Comments. Many meetings are unproductive because of poor preparation. In this section of the meeting review you can comment on issues such as, meeting outcomes (were the objectives realized?); deviations from the real purpose of the meeting; interruptions; the use of mobile phones in meetings; the effectiveness of the 'chair'; preparation and circulation of clear and accurate minutes; adherence to the agenda; decisions made and action points agreed; action points not processed by the next meeting; and actions resulting from the meeting.

5. Rank the importance of the meeting. Meetings are costly. So, at this point in the review you should make a decision about the importance of the meeting. Use a scale from one to five in order to decide whether the meeting is absolutely essential or useless to: a) the needs of the practice, hospital department, etc. and b) you personally. This information will help you to judge:
   • Is this meeting necessary?
   • Should I attend – always, occasionally or not at all?

For example, you might decide that there is an alternative to holding a meeting and the business can be conducted by correspondence or telephone.

All meetings should be reviewed in this way on a regular basis. This can be done as a group exercise among those people who need to meet regularly, but you can also do this alone as part of your personal time-management plan.

Time management – conclusion

People often describe stress as a feeling of being out of control. Effective time management enables you to take control of time and get control of your life. However, devotees of time management as a strategy for stress control have no illusions about the effort it takes initially. The only route is to 'take time' to 'make time' and to remember that there is a difference between being 'efficient' and 'effective'. Effectiveness is doing the right thing, whilst efficiency is doing the thing right – there is a difference! It is essential to have a written life plan with long- and short-term goals and an action plan. Use a diary and begin each day with a written plan or a to-do list – ideally scheduled and written the day before. Avoid becoming a workaholic and ensure that your diary is used to schedule your work, family and social activities. Do not feel guilty about taking some time out for thinking. We can easily become hypnotized into believing that anything other than action is time wasting. Certain skills can be learned and developed to help maximize the use of our time, such as speed-reading and report writing. Most people feel that they could perform better at work and make better use of their time – time management is a powerful tool to aid this process. Equally, the effective management of the workplace is also a useful stress-management strategy. This is the topic of the next chapter.

chapter FOUR

Creating an effective work environment

From the previous chapter we have seen that poor time-management skills can add to the burden of stress and pressure in the daily working life of the medical practitioner. Gaining effective control over one's immediate working environment is an extension of the time-management ethos. Therefore, in this chapter we consider ways of banishing workplace blues and creating a healthier place of work by managing the physical environment of the doctor more effectively.

Surveys conducted amongst GPs have indicated that a general dissatisfaction with physical working conditions exists (Sibbald et al. 2000). It would appear that satisfaction levels decreased between 1987 and 1990 (the survey conducted following the NHS reforms 1990), and by 1998 (the survey conducted by the National Primary Care Research and Development Centre) levels of job satisfaction had not recovered. This is a concern because job satisfaction is an important determinant of physician retention and turnover (Lichenstein 1998) and may also affect job performance (Grol et al. 1985). Since surveys have shown that GPs have reported increased stress levels associated with the working environment during the past decade, in this chapter we consider ways of improving the physical work conditions of the medical practitioner.

Typically, physicians tend to think that they do not have much control over their practices, but Childress (cited in Murray 2000) suggests that there is a range of things that they can control, including their finances, their health, their physical environment, how they manage their time and how their employees are trained. In this chapter we consider two aspects of the environment of the doctor and how stress is created, namely the:

- macro environment – that is, conditions of noise, heat, cold, ventilation and odours etc.
- micro environment – that is, the 'tangible' setting of an actual hospital ward, surgery or office.

Macro environment stress

In our physical surroundings, noise, lighting, heat, cold and odours are stimuli that bombard our senses and can affect our mood and overall mental state, whether or not we find the situation objectionable. Indeed, a considerable body of research has linked working conditions to mental health. Whilst much of this has focussed on the working conditions of the blue-collar employee, it is evident that poor mental health is directly related to unpleasant working conditions, the necessity to work fast and expend a lot of physical effort, and excessive and inconvenient hours (Kornhauser 1965).

In many hospital settings, and public sector buildings, lighting is usually artificial, monotonous, too bright or garish. Also, the windowless workplace of the hospital or surgery deprives us of natural daylight, a view of the world and the climate conditions outside. In addition to feeling isolated, poor lighting, or the flicker of ever-present fluorescent tubes can create eyestrain, damaged vision, visual fatigue, headaches, tension and frustration. Inadequate ventilation systems can worsen the problem of bad smells, even though health professionals often state that they seem to acquire immunity to them. However, attitudinal and physical problems can arise because a place of work is too hot, too cold, too draughty or too stuffy! It is also acknowledged that the subjective perception of thermal comfort is most important, and an inability to personally control one's physical work environment is a key factor in the perception of thermal comfort. The high level of noise in a busy casualty department, hospital ward or practice surgery can add to the level of pressure and strain experienced by the medical staff. Noise that is unpredictable and uncontrollable reduces one's overall perception of control over the environment and is often accompanied by a depressed mood. Indeed, change in noise levels, more than absolute noise levels, seems to be the irritant. Thus, an unexpected source of noise, like any other stressor, causes stress when it forces us to respond (Ivancevich & Matteson 1980). The main impact of excessive noise and similar stressors associated with our physical surroundings is to reduce our tolerance to everyday frustrations and to adversely affect motivation.

These forms of stress are actually described as *noise factors* because they take up the attentional capacity of the person and limit the ability to attend to task-relevant information. Job performance is likely to be impaired because we are unable to concentrate and social behaviour is adversely affected when we react by becoming irritable, hostile and less willing to help others. Although excessive noise (that is, 80 decibels or more) on a recurring, prolonged basis can cause stress, normal conversational speech of 70 decibels can also be disturbing and annoying, and cause the health professional to be less tolerant of the stressors intrinsic to the job itself. The need to work in an open-plan environment can exacerbate this type of stress.

Managing physical work conditions

General practice doctors are continually exposed to temperature and climate changes while on call, and are also exposed to the physical home environment of each patient. Doctors working in a hospital setting must practice in a building design dictated by architects, budgetary constraints and administrative processes. Thus, it might be difficult at first sight to understand what a doctor can achieve by including these sources of stress in a stress audit. However, stress-coping action is possible, so begin by completing a simple checklist to identify potential problem areas that could adversely affect your performance, well-being and health. For example:

- Is there sufficient light to perform the work well?
- Is the artificial lighting satisfactory? If not, why?
- Are noise levels high or disturbing?
- Is the workplace well ventilated?
- Are there any annoying draughts in the workplace?
- Is the temperature at work too low or too hot?
- Are there any dangerous situations in the work area?
- Are there any disturbing vibrations in the workplace?
- Are there any noxious odours in the workplace?
- Are the workplace hygiene standards satisfactory; for example, are work areas kept clean and free of risk of infection?

We believe that such issues should be addressed in the audit or psychological-risk-assessment process, because raising awareness about a potentially negative physical work situation or conditions, allows us to:

1. Gather non-emotive, objective data about potentially stressful physical work conditions and present this to the 'change-makers'. Thereby, it might be possible to bring about improvements to physical work conditions.
2. Examine the potential for gaining personal control – often it is possible to change certain aspects of the physical environment to reduce stress. Quite small changes can amount to significant improvements. For example:
   a. Is it possible to open the windows or, if not, try to go outside at regular intervals, because air conditioning dries out the mucus membranes in the nose and mouth that protect us against airborne germs. Keep

bottled mineral water close to hand and drink regularly to avoid dehydration. Use breaks to get some fresh air because it is charged with negative ions that reduce the fatigue and flu-like symptoms found in a stuffy workplace. If air is not circulating efficiently, you could experience a higher level of stress because too much carbon dioxide causes muscles to tense up.

b. Is it possible to move furniture in order to have an outside view – it might make you feel better about working in a dismal work area.

3. Examine faulty thinking about certain aspects of the physical environment. When we are in a state of stress we can often distort the reality of a situation, for example:

a. We might see things and judge them only in 'black or white'. An ability to view the 'shades of grey' of a situation helps us to avoid the problems associated with holding unrealistic expectations.

b. We often deny the real stress problem and seek something that appears to be 'respectable and safe' to blame as our source of pressure. For example, constant complaint, dissatisfaction and unhappiness about poor ventilation is 'safer' than accepting the reality of dealing with a bullying colleague or boss!

c. We jump to conclusions.

d. We magnify or exaggerate the situation.

e. We take things personally or over-generalize a situation. Instead of complaining that it is 'always' too stuffy and hot, an analysis might reveal that the work area is particularly unpleasant at certain times of the day. Therefore, if we cannot get help to rectify this problem, we might be able to plan our work schedule to be elsewhere at this time, or to find a task that is more conducive to the physically difficult or uncomfortable work environment.

f. We ignore important details.

By examining our irrational beliefs about our world we can avoid faulty thinking and move forward to deal with the actual stress problem. The process of challenging faulty thinking allows us to hold realistic expectations about a situation. It should be remembered that a state of stress only exists if we continue to hold unrealistic expectations about a situation, or believe that we do not have the ability to meet the demands created by that specific source of stress.

4. Identify what action, if any, can be taken in response to an identified source of stress. Our model of stress management provides us with three options, or levels of action, namely, primary stress management to eliminate the problem; secondary stress management to find ways to improve or optimize our response to the problem, and ensure that we do not respond in a negative or maladaptive way and thereby create more stress; and tertiary stress management in order to treat and take care of individuals who have become a casualty of exposure to stress.

For example, fluorescent lights constantly flicker and the brain registers this even if the eyes do not notice the effect. This acts as a stimulus that makes a constant demand on energy levels. Ideally, the replacement of fluorescent lights with full spectrum, natural daylight bulbs is a primary level action that is recommended to remove the stress of glare, eyestrain and constant exposure to artificial light. However, if a work area must remain windowless for hygiene, security or clinical reasons, and the need to work in artificial light, under fluorescent lighting cannot be removed, the job description of the employee should describe this situation. Also, medical staff that are required to work under these conditions should be advised of ways to avoid any health problems that might arise. In this instance, appropriate 'secondary level' stress-management strategies might include the provision of regular work breaks scheduled into the job; encouragement to use part of a lunch break to spend time outside of the building in natural daylight; regular eye examinations; and regular stress checks. Such actions would help to avoid the long-term negative effects of exposure to artificial lighting in a windowless work environment.

However, it is realistic to assume that certain conditions in the macro environment will be beyond our personal control. For example, it is rare that we work in a social vacuum, and so we must get along with other people. The diverse range of personnel working in a group-practice surgery or hospital department is unlikely to agree on an optimal temperature or ventilation conditions. This means that a compromise must be reached and negotiation skills will be needed to avoid stress in the physical work environment. Whilst it might be a challenge to make significant changes to our macro environment, there are aspects of the micro work environment that can be more easily managed to avoid stress at work.

Micro environment and stress

When we find ourselves confronted with a heavy and demanding workload, we can exacerbate the problem because we respond by putting on blinkers and stoically plodding through the volume of work. We need to take some time to question whether the work environment is conducive to such an intense level of activity. Time pressures and heavy demands tend to force us into this unsatisfactory work set-up, but we are unlikely to optimize our job performance and well-being if we continue to ignore certain aspects of the micro work environment.

Managing your work space

If you continually find that you misplace items; spend ages looking for documents; or fail to provide accurate information or paperwork to other health professionals, colleagues or administrative staff in a timely manner, then you might need to reorganize your work area in order to reduce stress levels, and become more effective. Our time-management teaching tells us that it is not enough to be efficient because it is possible that we might continue to work 'efficiently' on a task that does nothing to contribute to our performance 'effectiveness'. So, a plan for the re-organization of one's personal workspace must consider the issues of both effectiveness and efficiency. Although most now use computers for correspondence and record keeping, we are also guilty of remaining buried under a mountain of paper. We cling to old-fashioned filing cabinets, open shelving and overflowing drawers and shelves, because we do not take the time to organize ourselves. Too often we are guilty of behaving just like a hamster running in a wheel. We know that if we could stop running for a while and take some time to get more organized, life would be easier and probably more pleasant – BUT we dare not stop running!

Modernizing a drab work area might not be within the scope of your job, but making a complaint about the dirty conditions and windows, refusing to accept an uncomfortable chair, or cramped workspace might lead to improved conditions. You could try moving the furniture around to see if you can create a more productive and comfortable work environment. Most of us inherit a workspace from our predecessor and we tend to continue working under these same conditions without questioning whether it meets our personal needs, suits our style of working, or offers the most effective work arrangement. Take the blinkers off and take some time to ensure that your workspace is effective, efficient, pleasing and comfortable. Get out of a rut by moving the furniture around in your work area. Personal touches, such as discreet photographs, prints, or a vase of flowers can make a huge difference to a dismal or depressing work environment. Plants, for example the spider plant or peace lily, in the workplace can help to remove certain air pollutants.

Work smarter not harder – again!

It is suggested that an untidy work area is symptomatic of an untidy mind! A cluttered workspace does not necessarily lead to muddled thinking; it is the product of disorganized, muddled thinking originating from bad habits.

Clutter is bad for one's image and limits personal productivity. A cluttered situation usually arises because:

- we find it reassuring and comforting to have the things we need to hand. However, to other people this can project an image of insecurity and ineffectiveness
- we fear losing control of it if it is out of sight
- we believe, mistakenly, that leaving things readily available, just in case we need them, saves us time
- we believe that a desk piled high with work looks impressive and that other people will think that we are not working if we have a clear desk or work area.

In reality, these behaviours are counter-productive and the product of faulty thinking. They probably occur simply because we have not organized our work environment and do not know where to put the things we need. The truly muddled, cluttered individual probably does not have space to store things away because these are also cluttered and disorganized! A poorly managed work area also tends to be inefficient and uncomfortable. In addition, we run the risk of becoming overwhelmed because a task appears too daunting, or the clutter might trigger 'butterfly' behaviour as we respond to the sight of things and thereby react according to whim rather than our plan for the day.

To avoid this situation self-discipline is required. The following should be kept in mind:

- A desk or work area is for working AT, not for storing things ON.
- Clear your desk completely every night for security reasons and to ensure a fresh start the next day.
- You should have on your work area the papers or equipment needed for the current, active task. Everything else should be stored or filed away.
- Create a formal system where information, equipment or paper can be filed or stored. This system should be updated regularly. The use of coloured file covers or a colour code system can be used to indicate the various types of work, projects or work stages.

- Be ruthless about paper work and administrative demands – ask yourself if it is all really necessary or useful.
- It is more effective to use separate trays for your in and pending items. We are less likely to feel motivated or in control if we feel overwhelmed by a work tray that is full and overflowing.
- Maximize the use of computerized diaries, organizers and planners – but do keep in mind that these 'helper' tools can also create inordinately high stress levels until we discover how to use them and what they can do to help.
- Ensure that other people know and respect your method of working. This is very important when the work activity is based on a shift-work system, and the work area is open on a 24-hour per day basis. Let people know that you want to keep your work area tidy and explain where things should be stored or put in your absence. The use of a team building session is a useful way of negotiating conditions and a desirable, stress-free work environment that must be agreeable and shared by other people.

Stress, new technology and computers

Rapid technological development in the work environment has exposed medical practitioners to work 'with' and 'for' computers. We use communication tools such as the Internet, e-mail, voice mail and text messaging to stay in touch with each other. Whilst some people regard the need to be constantly and instantly available as a great source of stress, others bemoan a certain loss of personal contact as we communicate remotely for much of the time.

Computer information systems, decision support systems and tools such as word processors alter the ways that we perform our work. It has been suggested that technological advances aim to provide machines to deal with boring, repetitive, predictable and non-random activities and leave people to deal with important, unpredictable and random occurrences. However, the rapid pace of change and the constant need to keep up with new technology has generated 'techno-stress'. Whilst some doctors will admit to 'techno-stress' and a fear of computers, others have made a leap to the paperless office or surgery. But, as one doctor said:

I now work even later after surgery in order to update my computerised patient records so I can arrive the next day, to be reminded, by the computer when I switch on, that I need to write a repeat prescription for Mr XYZ!

The stress of work overload and the need to see ever more patients is a reality. Smith (2000) states that many doctors feel just like a hamster on the treadmill, and must run continually faster to stand still! He believes that the only way out of 'hamster healthcare' is to redesign healthcare by getting off the wheel, not running faster. One suggestion is to use information more creatively, particularly the Internet, to communicate with patients and manage the process of patient care as part of a fundamental redesign of clinical practice. In the USA (for example, Kaiser Permanente is committing a vast amount of funds – cited in Smith) and the UK (for example the Department of Trade and Industry Foresight Programme, 1999) ways of redesigning healthcare with the help of computer systems are currently being explored and include such concepts as virtual cyber physicians. Therefore, it is envisaged that the use of computers will assume a greater and more significant place in the future work environment of the doctor. So, love them or loathe them – computers seem to be here to stay in the medical practice workplace.

It might help to keep in mind that one does not need to know how a computer works in order to use one. Also, computers are not infallible, if you put 'rubbish' data in you get 'rubbish' results out. But, the use of certain computer software can also create diversion, relaxation and even humour while you are working. Whilst the 'paper-clip' office assistant might drive some of you crazy, it can also become a mental and visual diversion. Screen savers can also be soothing, relaxing and pure escapism! However, studies have shown that prolonged periods of computer use can create stressful work conditions and health problems. The following guidelines can be followed to reduce the physical strain and stress of working with computers:

1. Vary tasks to avoid holding a posture for lengthy periods. Sitting still at a computer can cause muscle tension, fatigue and discomfort, so change your posture regularly during the day.

2. Your computer monitor should be directly ahead so your eyes can look straight at the middle of the screen without bending your neck.

3. Use a chair that supports your lower back. Sit in a position that allows you to distribute your weight evenly without slouching or leaning forward towards the computer.

4. Sit with both feet on the floor – use a footrest to prevent your legs and feet from dangling.

5. Avoid bending or angling your wrists while typing. Keep the wrists straight and do not rest your palms on the work surface. A palm rest is to provide support during pauses, not while typing.

6. Check the height of your chair – you should be able to type with relaxed shoulders, with your elbows hanging at your side.

7. Take regular mini breaks – once every 15 minutes or so – look away from the monitor screen, into the distance, to avoid eye strain and poor eyesight. Blink your eyes regularly to protect the eyes. Blinking creates lubrication to prevent dryness of the eyes.

8. Have regular eye examinations.

9. Keep the monitor screen clean. Avoid glare and reflections on your monitor; use a desk-light rather than a central ceiling light if possible, or use a glare reduction filter or monitor visor.

10. Organize your work area to avoid overstretching for items in regular use.

11. Regularly stretch your arms and fingers, and rotate the shoulders. Physical activity is needed to avoid the

build up of lactic acid in the muscles as this causes muscles to become tense and painful.

12. Take breaks to relax and exercise:
    a. clench and relax muscles alternatively (neck, shoulders, arms, hands, legs).
    b. shrug shoulders, shake arms, stand-up and stretch – make sure you have room to stretch your arms and legs at your workstation
    c. if your job is sedentary, try to take breaks and walk briskly when possible
    d. take regular, moderate exercise; make sure your physical fitness is checked before embarking on a new fitness regime
    e. take deep breaths – intense concentration can cause shallow breathing.
13. Take meal breaks away from the work area; do not eat whilst working. Arrange to take a meal break with a friend or work colleague. An arrangement to lunch with someone else might help you avoid working through the day without taking a proper break.

In this chapter we have offered some simple ideas and basic guidelines for reducing strain and pressure in the work environment. We believe it is important to address these issues because the elimination of such stressors can either help to break a 'stress chain' or to prevent a stress chain from being formed. A source of stress rarely exists in isolation and one stressful condition can exacerbate another. For example, a noisy and uncomfortable work area is likely to make us less tolerant or effective when trying to deal with the demands of a difficult patient, or when interacting with work colleagues who do not appear to understand the urgency of our request. However, certain aspects of our own behaviour can create stress and this is the topic of the next chapter.

part THREE

Behaviour and stress

The quality of relationships plays a vital role in determining our health and well-being, and the workplace can offer opportunities to develop the social support networks that can protect us against the strains and pressures of modern-day living. Therefore, it is perhaps difficult to accept that we are capable of behaving in ways that can create stress to adversely affect our own personal well-being and cause problems for the people around us. Whilst we all believe that we have colleagues who frustrate and irritate us to the point of anger, our own style of behaviour can create unpleasant and stressful work conditions. Ultimately these bring both short- and long-term consequences for all parties concerned in terms of ineffective performance, poor productivity, ill health and poor psychological well-being. In addition to working with medical and support colleagues, doctors also find that they are working at what is known as, the 'boundary' of the organization (the group practice or hospital department) because they are required to deal with the sometimes difficult and problematic behaviour of patients, clients and the public as part of the job role. Since part of our strategy for the management of stress is AWARENESS, this section of the book aims to:

- increase our self-awareness about certain styles of behaviour as a mediator in our response to stress
- improve our understanding of the motivations underlying our actions that can lead to stress in the workplace
- consider effective strategies in eliminating or minimizing the negative impact of deleterious behaviours on performance, well-being and work–life balance.

In Chapter five we consider the links between stress and style of behaviour in terms of aggression, and in Chapter six we discuss the Type A styled behaviour of the doctor and the related issue of hostility. Before this, it is necessary to understand the basic principles of behaviour and why we continue to behave in ways that can cause harm to ourselves and the people around us.

Why do we behave in ways that create stress?

Although we will deal with only two basic styles of behaviour that are associated with the stress-prone personality, the following theory and principles provide an understanding of why we appear to continue to behave in ways that create and prolong stress. Essentially we behave according to five basic principles.

Behaviour is determined by its consequences

This premise is based on a theory originally described in 1951 by B.F. Skinner in an article for Scientific American, entitled, How to teach animals (Skinner 1969). He recognized that we are conditioned (i.e. our behaviour is shaped) to behave in certain ways by the consequences of our actions. So, if something nice happens as a result of our behaviour it is likely that we will continue to behave in the way that had immediately preceded this favourable outcome. Likewise, if something nasty is taken away as a result of our behaviour we also continue to behave in the way we did immediately prior to this desirable outcome. The reverse also applies, because we will cease our behaviour if something nasty occurs as a result of our actions or something nice is taken away. This, of course, is more commonly referred to as 'punishment'. These are known as the 'reinforcers' of behaviour. It is suggested that this is simply 'common sense psychology', because it means that people learn to behave in certain ways because they gain some form of reward or avoid behaving in ways that result in punishment or failure to gain a reward.

Behaviour that is rewarded will continue

If you continuously encounter a similar problem (that is, unwanted stress) at work, it is possible that some aspect of your own behaviour is causing this to occur. That is, a certain pattern of undesirable behaviour is being 'rewarded' in some way. Recognizing this by careful self-analysis and changing your *own* behaviour is the only way to avoid or prevent the problem reoccurring. For example, the difficult, audibly loud patient in the surgery reception area is often successful in the ploy of demanding to see a doctor 'now' because the practice staff will quickly try to remove themselves from this uncomfortable scenario by responding immediately. Therefore, the behaviour of the difficult patient is thus rewarded because they get what they want. Unfortunately, they will continue to behave in a similar way in the future to get urgent attention or simply to avoid waiting their turn like everyone else!

Behaviour that is punished or not rewarded will cease

This simple statement appears to lead us to the view that stopping undesirable behaviour only requires the administration of some form of punishment, or ensuring that the individual does not gain any benefit by behaving in an unwanted manner. Whilst the use non-reward might be an effective way of changing another person's behaviour, the use of punishment, even if it was possible, is rarely likely to work because we cannot fulfil the conditions that must exist.

Punishment must be immediate and occur every time

Punishment is only effective in changing behaviour when the behaviour is punished immediately after it occurs AND is punished every single time it happens. This explains why hangovers do not prevent us drinking to excess in the future – there is a DELAY between the pleasures of drinking alcohol in a social setting and the hangover on waking the following morning. Also, we do not ALWAYS have a hangover after a bout of drinking. Many health-related behaviour, such as smoking, overeating and the use of recreational drugs fit into this category. The pleasures are immediate, whilst the negative consequences are delayed. Unless the individual is strong-willed, the immediate consequences will exert most influence. The alternate healthy lifestyle that we all know we should adopt, is an example where the punishment is immediate but the rewards are delayed. Taking exercise for those who do not like it is an immediate punishment. The reward of a fitter body is delayed and so the influence of the immediate punishment will prevail (Sutherland et al. 2000). Therefore, there are only two appropriate strategies to use when seeking to change behaviour, but both of these require us to change our own behaviour.

Using positive reinforcement

In order to encourage the desired behaviour to occur more often, it is necessary to use positive reinforcement. This means:

- In a very specific way, identify the observable behaviour to be increased.
- Identify the reinforcer (also known as the reward) you intend to use. Not all people respond in the same way to reinforcers and so the main difficulty is

finding out what is effective for that particular individual. Smiles and praise are very powerful social reinforcers; special attention, privileges or increased opportunities to participate and take responsibility might also be effective.

- In order to ensure success, reinforcement should immediately follow the display of the desired behaviour.
- Initially it is appropriate to reinforce every display of the desired behaviour.
- When the new pattern is established it is possible to maintain the behaviour by changing to what is described as a 'variable ratio reinforcement schedule'. More simply put, it means that it is more effective to only reward the behaviour at variable times, rather than every time, because the individual knows that they will receive a reward (or pay-off) at sometime, and so they keep trying.

The use of non-reward

Non-reward means that you need to find a way of ensuring that the work colleague does not gain any benefit from their undesirable behaviour towards you. Non-reward leads to the cessation (or 'extinction') of the undesirable behaviour. It is not the same as ignoring the behaviour, rather that the work-colleague does not get any positive reward as a consequence. It means that you will need to change the way in which you relate to the person.

You cannot change another person's behaviour, only your own!

It is most important to acknowledge that to change the behaviour of another person, you first must change your own behaviour! From this we can begin to see why we behave in ways that create stress at work. In the next section we consider aggressive behaviour as a cause of workplace stress.

chapter FIVE

Aggression and stress

The aggressive individual always aims to win and it does not matter if this is at the expense of other people. It is generally agreed that we are behaving aggressively towards others when we assert our rights at the expense of others by dismissing or ignoring their basic rights. We might dismiss or ignore wants, needs, beliefs, opinions or feelings. Overt displays of aggression can become manifest in many different ways, taking both verbal and non-verbal forms. It must be remembered that a single, isolated incident of behaviour should be read in context, and alone cannot be taken as justification for applying the label of 'aggressive'. However, the following list describes aspects of aggression:

- Body position and movement – leaning forward towards another person; arms crossed high over the chest; hands on hips; unable to sit still; stride about; stand or sits in close proximity to other people, and tension.
- Position of head and facial expression – frowning; pressing lips tightly together; assuming a set facial expression; in the extreme, baring teeth; jutting the chin out and upwards.
- Eyes – using strong eye contact; maintaining a cold hard stare; piercing or glaring eyes; being last to look away in a conflict situation.
- Hands – precise, provocative hand gestures, such as the clenched fist; shaking of fist, or finger pointing and stabbing action.

- Voice – terse, abrupt and threatening speech; cold, loud voice; volume tending to rise at the end of sentences.

Characteristics of aggression

Below we describe some examples typical of aggressive behaviour. Are you guilty of behaving aggressively?

- Displaying a lack of interested in the opinions of other people.
- Constantly interrupting others with your opinion.
- Taking people for granted.
- Being short-tempered and resentful.
- Constantly finding fault in the work of other people.
- Tending to be critical and sarcastic.
- Being swift to jump to conclusions.
- Constantly feeling let down by others.
- Tending to be highly vocal – often shouting and swearing.
- Making decisions without consulting other people.
- Poking fun and devaluing the ideas of other people.
- Tending to overtly display displeasure.
- Being confrontational.
- Being quick to blame others.
- Saying exactly what you are thinking at the expense of other people.

Why we are aggressive

In simple terms, we are aggressive towards other people because there is an immediate pay off. We receive a reward for this style of behaviour and so the aggression continues. Aggressors get their own way because they ignore the rights of the other person. This usually means that the aggressor experiences a sense of power over other people. They can dominate and win.

An aggressive style of behaviour is often wrongly confused with assertive behaviour. It has been suggested that aggression is 'assertive' behaviour that has gone wrong. In fact, aggressive people usually believe that their approach is simply being honest and direct, and by 'straight talking' other people know exactly where they stand. Examination of the underlying beliefs of assertive, aggressive and non-assertive individuals indicates that we can conceptualize these behaviours along the following continuum.

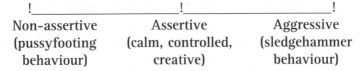

Non-assertive (pussyfooting behaviour)	Assertive (calm, controlled, creative)	Aggressive (sledgehammer behaviour)

Heron (1977) uses this model to describe the style of behaviour of an aggressive individual as the 'sledgehammer' approach, whereas the very non-assertive person is accused of 'pussyfooting'. Therefore, only when we behave in an assertive manner do we remain calm and controlled. By interacting in an assertive manner with other people we ensure a greater chance of communications being understood and accepted. It helps if we try to understand that the root causes of both aggressive and non-assertive behaviours seem to arise from the same core beliefs. That is:

- A belief that other people or situations are threatening.
- There is a failure to think rationally about one's self.
- There is an overreaction because of previous experiences; that is, displays of earlier non-assertion or aggression have not gone well or as expected.
- There is a failure to develop the skills of assertion.

Although the aggressor feels immediate and satisfying reward because they get what they want, in the long term they tend to experience feelings of regret, guilt or shame about the way in which they behaved. To appease this situation they might resort to apologizing in a profuse manner, try to make amends by being overhelpful or try to blame someone else for the situation. In such circumstances, self-esteem is likely to become damaged and anger is internalized. Also, use of aggression in response to a situation is energy demanding. The body is required to remain in a high state of physical and psychological alert and in the long term this causes problems associated with elevated blood pressure.

Consequences of aggressive behaviour in the healthcare work environment

Aggressive people tend to be regarded by colleagues as difficult, and a source of strain and pressure. They cause other members of staff in the medical practice to feel upset, angry, anxious and lacking in self-worth. Indeed, there is a growing awareness that oppressive behaviour is damaging to the well-being, morale, motivation and job performance of staff. Although the aggrieved will sometimes openly fight back or retaliate, in other circumstances, and more usually, they will suppress their feelings and may harbour a desire for revenge. Staff often find subtle ways of getting even, for example, by sabotage, failing to fulfil duties or some task that they had overtly been forced to agree to under duress. Clearly, neither overt conflict nor stifled hostility is productive workplace behaviour. The aggressive doctor who is a supervisor or manager of other people, who rules by fear, may ultimately suffer because personnel get even by underhanded means. Staff might appear to cooperate but resort to backbiting or delay tactics at every opportunity. Under extreme duress they will be quite happy to let an aggressive doctor 'dig their own grave' – and aid this process by letting a bad decision or mistake proceed to some ultimate bitter end. This might be the only way staff will be able to retaliate and be rid of a tyrant. Therefore, aggressive behaviour is costly when:

- performance deteriorates
- people quit
- personnel are frequently absent from work to avoid an aggressive doctor or work colleague
- poor quality decisions are made because staff fear speaking out and ideas are not fully discussed
- people leave because they are not prepared to tolerate working within an aggressive atmosphere. Also, it is likely that the people who stay will be the ones who react by 'keeping their heads below the parapet' in the hope of avoiding risky conflict behaviour. In this situ-

ation staff remain quiet about their concerns and voice few ideas. It means that levels of creativity are stifled and the individuals who would normally tender risky but better decisions are repressed

- it is possible that a powerful, aggressive doctor is often admired because they seem to get their own way and get things done. They become the role model for junior staff, thereby building and reinforcing an aggressive power culture within the workplace.

Dealing with aggression

A variety of techniques and strategies are available for dealing with aggressive behaviour including anger and conflict management, dealing with criticism and role negotiation.

In general terms it is important to remember to:

- remain focused on the specific issue and avoid emotional issues in an already heated situation
- refrain from making generalized comments or attack the individual's personality or attitude. This will certainly result in argument or denial since most people are likely to resent criticism or comment about their core functioning.

Anger and conflict management

Learning how to control our own anger and deal with it is very important in coping with the strains and pressures of the workplace. The inability to manage recurrent anger-provoking situations is associated with impulsive behaviours, aggression and cardiovascular disease. Suppressed anger is also viewed as maladaptive and is associated with cardiovascular problems.

Anger is defined as an emotional state that includes feelings of irritation, annoyance and rage, whilst aggression is a destructive behavioural response that is directed at others. Thus, anger can motivate aggression. When we become angry and distressed we cannot respond by fighting back since this is not socially acceptable behaviour in the healthcare environment, but neither can the doctor run away from the situation because there is a duty to fulfil job and role obligations. Losing control might cause you to lose your job or face disciplinary action. It will certainly cause you to lose the respect of other the people at work. To succumb to fight or flight can be psychologically damaging because we lose self-esteem and respect when we fail to master the anger-provoking situation. However, as we have suggested already, denial can cause us to experience frustration and stress-related psychosomatic disorders.

Understanding conflict

It is important to acknowledge that the human condition is fraught with conflict that is unavoidable in our modern-day lifestyle. Both society and the medical practice environment itself are filled with potential for conflict (for example, political instability and uncertainty; increasing crime rates; likelihood of divorce; the death of loved ones and patients; problem with patients and their families, with your own family and dependents; money worries; job reorganization, constant change to the job role, insecurity or threat of job loss). Therefore, it is more productive to expect that conflict will inevitably exist to disrupt, but it need not destroy.

Nevertheless, we need to acknowledge that not all conflict is bad. One cannot make an omelette without breaking eggs! It means that honest, openly expressed conflict, at the appropriate time, can be beneficial for our development and protect us from damage. Nevertheless, the suppression of emotions, the withholding of hostile feelings, and bottling anger up inside, can be damaging to our both our self-esteem and our heart. The individual who internalizes hostility and anger is at increased risk for heart disease and the mechanisms underlying the association between stress and heart disease are thought to relate to multiple and sustained increases in heart rate and blood pressure as a result of neuroendocrine activation (Steptoe et al. 1993), although individual differences in cardiovascular reactivity in response to acute stress are acknowledged (Carroll et al. 1991). Chronic psychological stress can provoke myocardial ischaemia in people who already have coronary artery disease, possibly by causing the endothelium in the coronary arties to malfunction. In this small-scale study in the UK, ten healthy men and eight men with non-insulin-dependent diabetes were asked to defend themselves to an audience against a spurious charge of shoplifting. The stress caused a measurable dysfunction in the healthy volunteers' vascular homeostasis that lasted for nearly 4 hours, and it was suggested that chronic stress of a similar magnitude could cause lasting endothelial damage (BMJ 2000, cited in Mineva).

Yet conflict is also beneficial since it can help us to break free of the bounds of convention and is, therefore, essential for creativity and innovation because it provides a spur to challenge, growth, development and change. We should keep in mind that 'functional conflict' works toward the goals of the medical practice, the healthcare team and the individual doctor, but 'dysfunctional conflict' blocks goal achievement, frustrates and irritates. There is nothing wrong with feeling angry when a patient, work colleague or boss lets you down, does not support your decisions or you when a situation gets tough, or acts in an inconsiderate way towards you. However, it is how you choose to behave and act on these feelings that is important in your work environment. Repressed anger over an extended period of time may be converted into elevated blood pressure, and so anger must be actively managed, not denied. Key Gilley (cited in Murray 2000) says:

Physicians are trained to push down the negative feelings, but at the same time they push away the love, joy and compassion, and enthusiasm. If you could take an ECG of physicians' souls, you'd see that most of them are flat-lining emotionally. We try to get them (in stress management seminars) to look at all the things that are scary, painful, or anger-provoking, and get them to unload all of it.

We differ in our orientation towards a conflict situation and five basic styles of behaviour can be identified. We will have a preference towards one of the following patterns of behaviour when we engage in a conflict situation:

1. Dominance – a desire to win in a conflict situation and overwhelm the other person.
2. Collaborative – this is a problem-solving approach since the individual has a desire to satisfy the wishes of all parties by finding an outcome that is acceptable to everyone.
3. Compromise – the individual is content if he/she gets part of their wants satisfied; this involves giving something to get something, usually by splitting the difference.
4. Avoidance – a low tolerance for conflict tends to force the individual to retreat from the conflict situation.
5. Accommodative – this is also known as 'non-assertion'; it is a 'smoothing' approach, whereby the individual tends to focus on the needs, wants and desires of the other person and ignores their own rights.

Understanding your orientation and the possible orientation of others involved in a conflict situation can help you manage an event more effectively. Finding a 'win–win' conflict reduction method should be your aim, unless you have decided that the conflict is in some way functional. Conflict is not automatically a negative experience since it creates constructive opportunities for discovering creative solutions. The identification of a superordinate goal (for example, a group-based incentive) which compels all parties in conflict to cooperate, because alone they cannot achieve the goal, is also a 'win–win' method of conflict reduction. 'Role exchange', that is, 'walking a mile in the other person's shoes', can also be a beneficial approach to resolving a conflict situation between two people or among groups and teams. However, both parties need to express a desire for change in the status quo.

Anger management

Anger is one of the commonest, most fundamental and most damaging of human emotions – it is a feeling or emotion. It is often a response to something that has happened and can be triggered by feelings of frustration, disappointment and injustice. Therefore, it is important that we express and release tension in a way that does not cause us damage, or harm to those around us. This can happen when anger leads to aggression. Anger is a natural and healthy response to stressful circumstances and may be helpful, for example, in getting motivated to tackle a problem or compete in sport. However, stored and suppressed anger can lead to high blood pressure, stomach ulcers and heart disease. In order to express anger and release tension in safety, we need to make sure that we have 'pathways' for protest in our work and home environments. Ideally, we should identify whom we can complain to. These people must be neutral observers.

As we have said, anger is a natural and healthy response, but some individuals become addicted to 'anger' and suffer the adverse impact of their angry behaviour. The following guidelines offer suggestions for an anger-management programme. The first phase is described as cognitive reparation and is needed to identify the anger-provoking situation. For example, the person is asked to:

1. Think about the difficult person who is arousing your anger
   a. Describe why they appear to be behaving in this way.
   b. How is the situation exacerbating the problem?
   c. What triggered the behaviour?
   d. Be honest – are you the cause of the anger?
   e. Describe how you reacted to the situation?
   f. Is this a common occurrence or a 'one-off' event with this person?
2. Acknowledge your feelings
   a. You feel angry – why?
   b. Are your feelings justified?
   c. Are *you* being aggressive in your anger?
   d. Do you feel in control or overwhelmed?
   e. Are you being realistic about the situation?

f. Are you jumping to conclusions?

In the second phase of this process the individual will learn and develop skills such as relaxation, communication techniques and cognitive control. In the final phase, the individual will use the new skills:

3. Stay in control

a. Remain calm and controlled.

b. Take a few deep breaths; breathe from the diaphragm and force your stomach muscles out to help you to breathe slowly and deeply; pause briefly to hold your breath before you exhale.

c. Controlled breathing will buy some thinking time and help you to delay your first utterance.

d. Use silent 'self-talk' to acknowledge how you are feeling; remember that some people will try to provoke you to anger because they find this situation rewarding. Acknowledging this will help you to stay in control of the situation.

4. Think about what you will do next

a. Ignore the situation or respond? If someone insults us, it is important to remember that we do not have to either defend or prove ourselves.

b. Decide what you want to get out of the situation.

c. Do you need more information before you can respond appropriately?

5. If you are going to respond, use assertiveness training techniques to say how you are feeling. Assertiveness is the capacity to influence or control other people without damaging the relationship. This means it is necessary to take account of others' interests and points of view (Galassi et al. 1981). Assertiveness is NOT about getting your own way at the expense of others.

a. Avoid the 'yes, but' approach because it causes the other person to 'dig in' their heels and defend their own position. An argument will be the most likely outcome of this tactic

b. Avoid being confrontational – remember, aggression is likely to breed aggression. Be specific and clear about what you are saying or asking. If you do not get a response to a request or question repeat it.

  c. Use empathy; this is the capacity to see another's point of view, to share their emotions and display this concern. It means actively listening to the other person, to show that you have heard what they are saying; that you respect them and take them seriously. This is not easy because your anger might drive you to speak your mind and ensure that the other person hears your opinion. Empathy means being able to put yourself in the other person's shoes and understand their feelings. It will allow you to speak about your feelings in a direct, positive manner and say clearly what you want to happen. For example, 'when you behave towards me like that, I feel . . . XX, and it has YYY effect on my behaviour. Can we (discuss/negotiate, etc)'

  d. If the other person is still angry it is often best to let them run out of steam before beginning a discussion.

  e. Make sure that your body language mirrors what you are saying.

6. Feelings of anger often develop because we feel that our basic human rights have been violated. Also, people might become angry with us because we have failed to allow others' their rights. The following are your rights, but they are also the rights of other people: You have the right to:

  a. be treated with respect as an intelligent, capable and equal person

  b. express feelings, opinions, needs and values

  c. say 'yes' and 'no' for yourself

  d. change your mind

  e. say, 'I do not understand'

  f. ask for what you want

  g. decline responsibility for other peoples' problems

  h. make mistakes

  i. deal with others without being dependent on them for approval.

7. Practise 'self-talk' (cognitive control) so you will be ready to deliver the right response and cope when your anger is provoked.

   a. Master and overlearn phrases to use in maintaining control when you feel you are becoming angry.

   b. Use visual imagery to imagine yourself behaving in a controlled way when provoked.

8. Alter the way you relate to the other person by being assertive rather than becoming aggressive or non-assertive. Ultimately it means that you refuse to allow another person to control your behaviour.

9. Medicine is often viewed as a macho male-dominated culture, and macho males do not dance, eat quiche or complain – instead they quietly implode (Cejka 1999). According to Denning (cited in Murray 2000) there is still a lot of that, 'I-eat-stress-for-breakfast' machismo out there, especially among surgeons. He suggests that they are slow to seek help, if they seek it at all! Thus there is a need to break this damaging mould, to seek help and to give voice to pent-up emotions. You can reduce stress by sharing your feelings with a colleague or partner, or blow off steam and hear yourself talk before a willing audience (the topic of 'venting steam' is discussed further in the final chapter).

Anger can be physically, mentally, socially and economically damaging to all parties involved. The strains and pressure of the workplace can create anger-producing situations, but it is essential that we manage the response to minimize harm to health, well-being and relationships at work and at home.

Dealing with criticism

We can avoid anger and becoming angry if we learn how to give and receive criticism. The following guidelines will help to reduce the pressures that we experience when both giving and receiving criticism. There are five key points to keep in mind:

1. Remain calm
2. Stay positive

3. Be objective
4. Use brief, clear statements
5. Be constructive.

When you are criticized, it may help to remember the following points:

- When a personal attack is made on you, the only productive way of dealing with this is to be assertive. By resorting to aggressive or non-assertive behaviour the situation will become worse and the outcome will be unfavourable. You have the right to ask the other person not to personalize an attack
- Other people have a right to criticize you but they do not have the right to put you down or humiliate you in front of other people.
- If you become angry, annoyed or scared, you will probably fail to listen to what is being said during the interaction and might react inappropriately. Relax and take a few deep breaths. This will prevent you from speaking too soon and ensure that you are clear about what is being said about your behaviour or performance.
- If the criticism is vague or ambiguous, you have the right to ask the person to be more specific and quote examples.
- Make sure that you are not guilty of faulty thinking when either giving or receiving criticism. Use self-talk to examine potentially damaging thoughts. Faulty thinking errors include over-generalizing from one event to another; exaggeration; minimization; black and white thinking; holding unrealistic expectations; and irrational assumptions. Ask yourself if the criticism is justified and fair?
- When receiving criticism it is helpful to state the criticism in your own words. Use of reflection, or 'active listening' ensures that both parties are clear about what is being said. It shows the other person that you understand the criticism.
- When you are criticized you must ask if the judgement is valid. By acknowledging criticism and asking for further information, you can use the criticism to

good effect. If the criticism is done badly and your feelings are hurt, it is appropriate to state this in an assertive way. Begin by using the technique of reflecting back what was said to you before stating your feelings. This ensures the other person realizes that you have understood the criticism, rather than assuming that you are going to start an argument or disagree.

When you wish to direct criticism at another person, use the following guidelines:

- Criticism should be directed at the behaviour that we find stressful, and is having a negative impact on our own behaviour, performance or well-being, rather than towards the personality or attitude of the other person.
- Be specific when giving criticism; encourage the other party to respond to you and then move forward by making and agreeing suggestions for future action. Try to find something positive to say first, but be genuine. Otherwise do not attempt it! Avoid putting the other person in a defensive position by blaming. For example, the wrong way to approach a situation is to say, 'You are absolutely useless – this is the wrong documentation again. Get it right or there will be trouble!' Compare this to, 'I want to talk to you about the documentation required for X. This is the second time that you have given me the wrong forms. Do you know why this is happening? (wait for a response). How can we avoid this occurring again?'
- When you complain, explain how you feel and why and then stay quiet in order to allow the other person to respond. Resist the urge to relieve your tension by continuing to talk. It is an important part of the technique to let the other person feel some pressure in order for them to be able to take responsibility, cooperate and act on your complaint.
- If you face outright hostility you can diffuse the situation by stating how you think the other person is feeling, rather than respond by trying to defend yourself, since this latter strategy is more likely to cause an argu-

ment. For example, say, 'Something has clearly upset you. I am sorry about that', or 'I am very surprised to hear you say that. Something has clearly upset you.'

- Avoid sarcasm – it shows a lack of respect and implies contempt. Also, people might not be quite sure what you are getting at when they do respond; they also risk being accused of having no sense of humour or being too sensitive.

- Summarize what actions have been agreed to ensure that both parties are clear about the outcomes. Since the interaction can be heavy with emotion, it is easy to deny or fail to acknowledge the outcome if it is not clarified. Also, the pace of this type of dialogue can move very fast and develop into an argument if one or the other individual fails to adopt an assertive approach. Stay calm, control your breathing and speak slowly and quietly to avoid escalation of the situation.

Role negotiation

Role negotiation is a useful technique to use when an individual is unwilling to change because it might mean a loss of power or influence. Roger Harrison (1974) suggests that this method works because most people prefer a fair negotiated settlement to a state of unresolved conflict. So, they will be motivated to engage in some action themselves and make concessions in order to achieve this aim. In role negotiation the change effort is focused solely on the working relationships among the people involved and the likes and dislikes for one another in the relationship are avoided. Again, the personal feelings of the people involved are avoided. It is necessary to create a structure in which a controlled interaction can take place. Each person involved discusses and agrees in writing to change certain behaviours, in return for changes in behaviour by the other party. For example:

1. Each person asks for changes in the behaviour of the other party to allow them be more effective at work, in exchange for changing some aspect of their own behaviour. This should also serve to improve the effectiveness

of the other party involved. It means an accurate understanding of the issue is vital.

2. It is crucial to avoid generalities and be specific. For example, you ask the other person to:
   a. stop doing 'X'
   b. do more of 'Y'
   c. do less of 'Z'.

3. In return, these are the type of actions that the other person will ask of you.

4. All requests and agreements must made be in writing.

5. Each person must give something in order to get something. That is, 'If you do "X" I will do "Y"'.

6. If one party reneges on their part of the bargain, the whole contract becomes invalid.

This technique can be used between individual doctors, within a practice group, to negotiate among the members of a healthcare team, or between a doctor manager and the healthcare team. A facilitator tends to be used for optimal effectiveness. Some progress follow-up is required to determine whether the contracts are being honoured

Summary – managing aggression

It is important that aggression is diffused without resorting to aggression and anger in yourself. Coping with aggression is demanding and it is often easier in the short term to retaliate with either an aggressive or non-assertive response. However, it is unlikely that you will be happy about this outcome in the long term. So, it is worthwhile to persevere and try to actively manage your aggressive tendencies or the aggression of a colleague or patient. In summary:

1. Gain control of your thoughts and feelings by breathing correctly. This buys you some time to slow down the fast pace of an aggressive interaction.

2. Pause and then ask for information to ensure that you understand the situation. Encourage the aggressor to talk about the feelings that are causing their behaviour.

3. Check your own inner dialogue for faulty thinking; are you harbouring unrealistic or irrational beliefs?

4. Use empathetic listening to show the other person that you understand what they are saying, and that you respect them and take them seriously.

5. Clarify discrepancies that exist. Aggression often arises from misunderstandings.

6. Explain how you are feeling and the impact of the anger on your actions.

7. Offer alternative solutions to the problem.

8. Try to see points in the other person's argument with which you can agree.

9. If aggression is maintained, cease interactions with the person by leaving the situation.

10. Use the broken record technique to refuse a request, to get someone to listen to you or your ideas, or to get a message across. You simply repeat your message, over and over again, in a calm way until it is received.

11. Do not be afraid to use the power of silence. It will help you to gain control in an aggressive interaction.

12. Practice saying 'no'.

13. Use the fogging technique to diffuse an aggressive interaction. This approach allows you to recognize what is happening without agreeing with it so that you do not become either defensive or aggressive. You are not required to back-down or agree with the attack. For example, if a colleague says, 'You handled that patient ineffectively and acted in a weak way by letting them get away with it', You might say, 'Yes, I can see that you feel I acted in a weak manner'.

The feelings that people call stress have been described as tension, worry, panic, frustration, doubt, confusion, depression, fear or insecurity. Thus stress is the emotional product of work and living in contemporary society. Likewise, anger is an emotion that can give rise to aggression, with negative implications for the performance, effectiveness and well-being of the medical practitioner. Since the workplace requires a considerable degree of emotional constraint, it is worthwhile learning how to deal effectively with aggression. It is a learned behaviour and so it can be altered. However, this requires commitment, patience and a well-structured plan. In the next chapter we discuss the style of behaviour known as Type A coronary-prone behaviour. This is another of the stress-prone personality types who appear to create stress for themselves and the people who work with them.

chapter SIX

Type A behaviour and stress

In the 1950s, cardiologists Meyer Friedman and Ray Rosenman described a certain pattern of behaviour among heart attack survivors that became known as Type A behaviour (Friedman & Rosenman 1974). An absence of Type A characteristics is referred to as a Type B style of behaviour. In this chapter we describe this style of behaviour, explain how and why it is implicated in the stress process, provide a questionnaire for the self-assessment of the Type A behaviour style, and offer stress-management guidelines for Type A doctors. After many years of research it is now acknowledged that this style of behaviour is a risk factor for heart disease, independent of heredity and factors, such as high blood pressure and high levels of cholesterol, cigarette smoking, alcohol consumption and obesity. However, recent research suggests that it is the hostility and 'anger-in' (internalizing anger and irritation with self and other people) components of Type A behaviour that are likely to be the factors that increase the risk of diseases of the heart. The inability of Type A individuals to relax easily may explain their more frequent use of alcohol, the increased hostility and social aggression observed, and the risk of heart disease. Their active style of behaviour might be a contributory factor in the higher physiological reactivity observed (or vice-versa?), since studies have shown that, when challenged to perform well on a task, Type As respond with higher increases in heart rate, catecholamine levels and blood pressure than Type Bs. Also, after exposure to a stress situation, Type As exhibited greater platelet aggregation and raised serum cholesterol levels. Therefore, it is suggested that it is the style of behaviour of the Type A person that makes them stress prone and a source of stress for other people.

Measuring Type A behaviour

You can use the following questionnaire to classify your style of behaviour and temperament. An absence of the Type A behavioural characteristics is called Type B behaviour. Circle one number for each of the statements that best reflects the way you behave in your everyday life. For example, if you tend to be prompt for appointments, you might want to circle a number between 7 and 11. If you tend to be more casual about time keeping you would circle one of the lower numbers, between 1 and 5.

The higher the score the more firmly your behavioural style can be classified as Type A behaviour. By placing a score along the continuum at the bottom of Table 6.1 you can see if you lean more towards one style of behaving rather than the other. Eighty-four is the mid-point score and anyone scoring above that is inclined towards Type A, and anyone below inclines more towards Type B behaviour. Type A behaviour is a multifaceted personality trait, therefore certain situations might illicit a variation in the way in which you respond. Nevertheless, the Type A individual is usually able to identify their proclivity towards the characteristic Type A behaviour if they answer truthfully. However, as a Type A you are also likely to deny these tendencies and so it might be beneficial for someone who knows you well to also complete a copy of this questionnaire and rate their perceptions of you, with the purpose of comparing the two responses. This might provide a more accurate picture of your Type A tendencies.

Table 6.1   A measure of Type a Behaviour

Style of behaviour	Rating Scale	Style of behaviour
Casual about appointments	1 2 3 4 5 6 7 8 9 10 11	Never late
Not competitive	1 2 3 4 5 6 7 8 9 10 11	Very competitive
Good listener	1 2 3 4 5 6 7 8 9 10 11	Anticipates what others are going to say – nods, attempts to finish for them
Never feels rushed – even when under pressure	1 2 3 4 5 6 7 8 9 10 11	Always rushed
Can wait patiently	1 2 3 4 5 6 7 8 9 10 11	Impatient while waiting
Takes things one at a time	1 2 3 4 5 6 7 8 9 10 11	Tries to do many things at once, thinks about what will do next
Slow, deliberate talker	1 2 3 4 5 6 7 8 9 10 11	Emphatic in speech – fast and forceful
Cares about satisfying him/herself no matter what others may think	1 2 3 4 5 6 7 8 9 10 11	Wants a good job recognized by others
Slow doing things	1 2 3 4 5 6 7 8 9 10 11	Fast – eating, walking etc.
Easy – going	1 2 3 4 5 6 7 8 9 10 11	Hard-driving – pushing yourself and others
Expresses feelings	1 2 3 4 5 6 7 8 9 10 11	Hides feelings
Many outside interests	1 2 3 4 5 6 7 8 9 10 11	Few interests outside work/home
Unambitious	1 2 3 4 5 6 7 8 9 10 11	Ambitious
Casual	1 2 3 4 5 6 7 8 9 10 11	Eager to get things done

Add your scores

Score = _____

Plot your score below

Type B   Type A

| |_____|_____|

14   84   154

Source: Cooper's adaptation of the Bortner Type A Scale

Characteristics of Type A behaviour

Research evidence suggests that in some instances the Type A style of behaviour might be deleterious to both the individual and business success. The following list of Type

A behaviour characteristics helps us to understand how these individuals can create and exacerbate stress both at work and at home. Type As:

- tend to be devoted to work and work long hours
- usually feel guilty when they are not working or are relaxing
- take work home evenings and weekends
- have a chronic sense of time urgency; they always seem rushed and work under impossible deadlines – usually self-imposed
- feel a constant need to hurry which is reflected in their overt behaviour since they usually walk, talk, and even eat rapidly, in fact, Type A behaviour is also known as 'the hurry disease'
- use emphatic gestures such as banging the fist on a table, or fist clenching and waving; these outbursts occur because they become frustrated with their own efforts, and thwarted goals, *and* with the efforts of those who work with them
- feel misunderstood by their immediate boss
- attempt to schedule more and more in less and less time; they make few allowances for unforeseen events
- often attempt to do two or more things at the same time; this is known as 'polyphasic activity'; for example, the typical Type A doctor will want to read while eating; apply make-up or use an electric razor while driving the car, or continue to work on patient records while talking on the telephone about a completely unrelated event!
- hate being kept waiting, particularly in queues
- tend to finish sentences for other people, or frequently urge them to the point by interspersing the dialogue with, 'yes, yes, yes', or by repeating, 'uh huh' over and over again
- frequent sighing is a typical Type A trait
- the Type A speech pattern reflects underlying aggression or hostility since they adopt the habit of explosively accentuating various key words into ordinary

speech without any real need; they often have a strong voice and speech is clipped, rapid and emphatic; and the last few words of sentences are rushed out as if to quicken the delivery of what they want to say, thereby exhibiting impatience, even with themselves

- find it difficult to talk about anything other than work-related interests and perhaps do not have any interests outside of work to discuss with others
- rarely take all their holiday entitlement or cut holidays short; they really believe that the medical practice cannot function without their presence!
- rarely notice things (or people) around them in the workplace that are not related to the task or the means of getting the job done
- are very competitive with themselves and everyone around them; they constantly set themselves (and other people) goals that they continually strive to better – since Type A doctors drive themselves to meet high and often unrealistic standards, it is not surprising that they feel angry when they fail to achieve these goals or make a mistake – they feel frustration and become easily irritated when they experience failure
- exhibit a strong need to be in control of events around them; a perceived lack of control over events will cause the Type A doctor to become even more extreme in their time-urgent, and hasty behaviours.

Why we behave as a Type A

Type A behaviour seems to be a response to challenge in the environment. As we have noted, by engaging in active coping in threat situations the Type A doctor remains physiologically aroused. Whilst some researchers have tried to claim a heritability component to Type A behaviour, it is more likely that the behaviour is learned. Indeed, it must be a way of coping which the Type A individual finds rewarding in some way in order for the behaviour pattern to continue. Whilst the Type A coronary-prone behaviour pattern might be costly to a healthcare business in the long term, the immediate outcome is often one of gain for these workaholic doctors. Thus, Type As are both tolerated and rewarded with promotion and privilege for their actions and so their behaviour pattern is reinforced (that is, rewarded). The Type A doctor is likened to Sisyphus, King of Corinth who was condemned to roll a huge marble block up a hill. As soon as it reached the top, it rolled down again and Sisyphus immediately began the task again. This striving against real or imagined odds, irrespective of the outcome, along with an inability to enjoy the satisfaction of achievement or relaxation, was the way in which Wolf (1960) described the coronary-prone Type A person.

The consequences of Type A behaviour at work

Whilst the Type A doctor is highly sociable, they can create stress because of their constant need to compete and never be defeated. They tend not to listen or let you finish what you want to say, often because they believe they already have the correct and perfect solution to the problem. Indeed, they tend to think they are always right. Type A work colleagues are usually not interested in anything else outside of the medical work environment and as peers they are unlikely to be supportive of each other. They also tend to be poor team players because they do not want to share success or work towards a common goal. In fact, they rarely take any personal interest in the immediate work environment or the people around them. The Type A doctor also appears to react adversely to highly structured work settings that place strict controls over their activities. They tend to suppress subjective states and deny the physical effects of fatigue and strain. Thus, by their own actions, the Type A individual creates stress for themselves and other people. Working for a Type A doctor is often a strain because they demand and maintain a strict control over what is going on. The Type A doctor often finds it quicker to do a job rather than take time to show someone else what to do. Thus, they fail to develop staff or delegate effectively. This explains why their workload is so high and the constant overload pressure makes them irritable and hostile. The Type A doctor is rarely satisfied with the efforts of their staff and constantly expects everyone else to work to their demanding pace. Ultimately everyone suffers the consequences of the dysfunctional behaviours of the workaholic, perfectionist and Type A doctor.

Managing your Type A behaviour

If you have identified your style of behaviour as Type A rather than Type B, the following suggestions might be helpful in minimizing the potentially damaging elements of this style of behaviour.

1. Type A individuals are not good listeners and tend to speak for others. They even finish sentences for other people. To restrain yourself from being the centre of attention by constantly talking; force yourself to listen to other people by remembering the axiom, 'we have two ears, but only one mouth – use them in these proportions!' Ask yourself:
   a. do I really have anything important to say?
   b. does anyone want to hear it?
   c. is this the time to say it?
2. Thank or reward people for their efforts.
3. Control obsessional, time-directed, activity. Type A individuals are bad at estimating the amount of time they need to complete tasks or make journeys. Since you exhibit this tendency, work out the time you think you need, and then add on some extra time – at least 10 minutes. This might help to prevent you from driving in a 'white-knuckle' manner from place to place, or going through traffic lights on 'deep amber'. Make sure you always carry something to read, so if you arrive early for an appointment you will not become impatient because you feel you are wasting time. Ultimately you should aim to sit, relax, and absorb the environment around you while you unwind and mentally prepare yourself for the work activity. However, this strategy might initially create too much stress for the Type A

individual. So, gradually build up your tolerance for being kept waiting by deliberately exposing yourself to situations where this is likely to happen. Use 'self-talk' (see PART FOUR) to ensure that you do not become impatient or angry. Try to smile, look around and 'take time to smell the roses'. Think about something pleasant that is going to happen soon and make sure that you reward yourself for controlling your time-directed behaviour.

4. Do not try to do several tasks at once!

5. Remember, not all duties require your immediate attention or action. A slower, more deliberate response and pace might lead to better results, or an improvement in your quality of decision making. When you feel under pressure, ask yourself, 'Will this matter or have any importance 5 years from now?' or, 'Must I do this right now – can I take some time to think about the best way of accomplishing the task'. It is vital to accept that a successful life is always unfinished. Life must be structured around uncompleted tasks and events – only a corpse is completely finished!

6. Reduce your workaholic tendencies by engaging in social activities outside of work. Do not succumb to interests that foster hard driving, achievement oriented, impatient behaviours. If the activity creates feelings of hostility, anger or irritation, do not do it! For example, if you have just thrown your second set of golf clubs into the lake because your performance has not improved this season, then golf may not be a hobby for you. Try to engage in activities that provide satisfaction and help you to stay calm, without triggering your natural Type A competitive tendencies. The aim is to establish a realistic balance between professional- and personal-life activities and achievements.

7. Avoid setting unrealistic goals and deadlines for yourself and other people.

8. Cease trying to be such an idealist, particularly if it creates disappointment or hostility towards others.

9. Do not internalize anger or irritation. This style of coping is extremely damaging. Find ways to 'vent steam'

(see the final chapter), for example, by engaging in vigorous physical activity; write that 'angry' letter – keep it somewhere safe until you calm down and can read it again, before deciding on the best course of action; or talk to trusted friends or a colleague about your anger, fears and anxieties.

10. Learn to say 'no' in order to protect your time. Stop trying to prove yourself!

11. Avoid working for long periods of time without taking a break or breathing space since this is not an effective work strategy. A break away from work helps to take the pressure and tension out of the task and refreshes you ready for action again. Get completely away from your work area and engage in something that is not related to the task. Ensure that you take work breaks and a proper lunch break, preferably in the company of colleagues. Type As often think that time spent in social intercourse is wasted time, when in fact, they should accept that time spent this way is well spent. Type A doctors need to develop social relationships as a buffer against the strains and pressures created by their style of behaviour. This is explained in more detail in the final chapter on social support as a stress-coping strategy.

12. Monitor the number of times a week you are the first person to arrive and the last person to leave the place of work. Is this behaviour really necessary? Resolve to arrive last and leave first at least twice during the week.

13. Take all your holiday entitlement and ensure that your colleagues and staff follow your example.

14. Take regular exercise – you will have higher energy levels and feel mellower if you incorporate regular physical activity into your life.

15. Learn and use some form of relaxation. We have suggested that Type A doctors need to learn to relax more. Strategies and guidance for this are included in the last chapter of this book.

16. Do not expect to completely change your behaviour from Type A to a Type B style. This is an unrealistic

and impossible goal. Trying to encourage the hare to move around just like a tortoise is evolutional suicide – just ask the fox! Recognize and accept your limitations, and gradually begin to take more control of your drive to be Type A.

17. Get off the hot seat for a while. If you are suffering from burnout (see Chapter three) the need to take a career break or sabbatical is important (see the final chapter). Even those who are 'smouldering' rather than burned-out might benefit from a job change or a downshift in career on a temporary or permanent basis. Whilst most of us might question the financial and professional sanity of such a decision, the Type A habit of ignoring the physical and psychological symptoms associated with strain and pressure could, in the long term, exert a cost that is too high or too final!

Type A behaviour: conclusion

It would seem that we learn to become Type A in response to the healthcare work environment. Whilst the study of GPs reported by Sutherland and Cooper (1992) found that GPs displayed similar Type A behaviour tendencies to the general population, it was also apparent that Type A doctors were more anxious and depressed than their Type B counterparts, irrespective of gender. Type As appeared to be overly conscious of time, very ambitious, hard driven and competitive. The evidence suggested that this is not good for doctors or the patients they treat. In a study of 1176 healthcare workers in the UK, Rees and Cooper (1992) found that the hospital doctors scored higher on a measure of Type A behaviour than their counterparts working as nurses, in professions allied to medicine in scientific and technical jobs, as ancillary workers, or in administrative and clerical jobs. However, although they were more likely to be Type A, these doctors reported higher levels of job satisfaction than their co-workers. They also tended to feel 'in control' compared to the other groups in this study, but were less likely to use social support as a stress-coping strategy. This is important, because the Type A individual has a strong need for control, and when this becomes thwarted for any reason, stress levels also become elevated to a dangerous degree. Other research findings indicate that at certain times we become more Type A in our style of behaviour. For example, it is was noted that junior house doctors were significantly more Type A in behaviour at the end of their first year in a hospital, than they were during training at medical school.

Thus, if we can learn to become Type A, we can learn to manage the potentially deleterious aspects of this style of behaviour. It is not easy to change, but it is preferable to tackle our stress-prone tendencies before irreparable harm is caused. In the next and final part of the book we provide specific advice about relaxation techniques and ways of developing social-support networks for Type A doctors together with other useful options for the management of stress. These, of course, are not restricted to the Type A doctor. Indeed, as we have seen in earlier chapters, there is not one stress problem and neither is there one solution. In addition, we all differ in our preferred ways of coping. Thus, a smorgasbord of stress-management techniques is offered in the next section to help the doctor build and develop a personal plan for the effective management of stress and pressure.

A stress-management strategy

The recommended approach to stress management has been described as the 'Triple A' model. Stress management is effective when we:

- increase our understanding and AWARENESS about the nature of stress at work and the negative impact of mismanaged stress
- identify stress through the process of ANALYSIS or diagnosis
- take ACTION that is guided and informed by the process of awareness raising and analysis.

In PART ONE we explained the stress process, how and why it can be harmful to doctors, and ways of identifying mismanaged stress. In PARTS TWO and THREE we offered guidance on stress-management options for medical practitioners. We advised that stress levels are effectively reduced and controlled by creating a more effective work environment, and by developing and improving time-management skills. In addition, the links between certain styles of behaviour and stress were explained together with ways of reducing the strains typically experienced by these stress-prone personalities. In this final part we present an overall strategy for the management of stress and guidance on specific stress-management techniques for doctors and their immediate staff.

chapter SEVEN

A twelve-point personal plan

As we have seen, work-related stress and the overspill of problems from the work to the home environment create physical, psychological, emotional and behavioural problems for doctors and the people who work and live with them. However, we are all unique in our response to stress and our preferred coping style and so will respond to stress in different ways. A wide range of factors can create unwanted pressure or stress. Stimulating pressure will change to debilitating stress when the medical practitioner feels unable to cope, becomes anxious or insecure about such feelings, and begins to adopt negative coping behaviours that, in the long term, simply become an additional source of strain. Thus, it is important that the doctor is able to correctly identify a source of stress and take the appropriate action. The following twelve-point plan is offered as a self-management approach to the management of stress.

1. Identify the sources of pressure in your life – know thyself. Learn to recognize your stress reactions:
   a. keep a stress log or diary
   b. analyze and pinpoint the sources of stress and stress agents; can you bring about a change?
2. Tackle the cause of your stress. Although we would advocate the use of relaxation techniques, controlled breathing and positive thinking as an approach to the management of stress, it is also necessary to try to actively deal with

the cause of your strain and discomfort. It is more beneficial to sit down with the 'difficult' colleague, who is the cause of your perceived problem and try and negotiate a solution. Perhaps they did not realize the consequences of their actions or, after a discussion, you may understand why they are behaving towards you in this way. Alternatively, you might need to accept that you both must alter your behaviour towards each other to resolve the problem. So, rather than just counting to ten while breathing deeply, make sure that you are in control of the situation and then ask the individual if you can meet to discuss a problem that you are having, and which involves them. By keeping a stress log and reviewing your entries, it is likely that you are able to find ways to take the 'heat' out of a difficult situation. For example, a work overload problem might be eliminated if you have kept a time log. The information can help you to decide if you are able to delegate some of the work to someone else, or you are doing a task that does not serve any purpose because the system has changed and you are simply duplicating something already covered elsewhere.

a. To delegate successfully, you must acknowledge and control your workaholic, perfectionist tendencies by asking for help.

b. Remember, a stress reaction is a warning – so take action. You might need to remove yourself from the source of stress if you cannot remove it. For example, take a break from the task, take a holiday, change your job, get professional help, and see your own doctor!

c. Your stress log will help identify your tendency to feel stressed by minor issues or things that are soon forgotten. It is easy to get into the bad habit of overreacting to the small stuff. This can drain your energy reserves. So, do not create obsessions about small worries. Do not torment yourself with the 'what ifs' – react to the hazard, not the threat!

3. Clarify and set personal and career goals. Set 'SMART' goals. This means that they should be, specific, measurable, achievable, realistic and time-bounded. This is important advice for the doctor with workaholic tendencies and the Type A behaviour prone individuals. It is also recommended that you produce a written life-plan.

   a. Develop and write a plan with 1-year, 3-year and 5-year marker points, objectives and action strategies. That is, identify and describe briefly what you are going to do, when and how.

   b. Next, establish priorities for both work- and home-life goals. Classify your goals as follows and assign a time-line to each:

      i. As – must do

      ii. Bs – would like to do

      iii. Cs – not essential.

   d. Monitor your progress by frequently examining your plan. However, your plan should be a guide and helper, thus you should avoid becoming a slave to a plan.

   e. Reward success and examine the failures – learn from them and then move on. Do not constantly punish yourself or resort to maladaptive and damaging ways of coping if you have not reached your goal. Instead, try to understand the reasons for not achieving a specific goal.

   f. Make a copy of the following reflections from this 87-year-old lady, Nadine Stair from Louisville, and display them somewhere prominently. She said, '**I'd pick more daisies** – if I had my life to live over, I'd try to make more mistakes next time (perhaps not medical mistakes!). I would relax. I would limber up. I would be sillier than I have been this trip. I would be crazier. I would be less hygienic. I would take more chances. I would take more trips. I would climb more mountains, swim more rivers and watch more sunsets .... I would eat more ice-cream and less beans. I would have more actual troubles and fewer imaginary ones. You see I am one of those people who live pro-phylactically and sanely and sensibly, hour by hour, day by day. Oh, I've had my moments and, if I had to do it all again, I'd have more of them. In fact, I'd try to have nothing else. Just moments – one after another – instead of living so many years ahead each day. I have been one of those people who never goes anywhere without a thermometer, a hot water bottle, a gargle, a raincoat and a parachute. If I had to do it again, I would go places and do things, and travel lighter than I have. If I had my life over, I would start bare-footed earlier in the spring and stay that way later in the fall. I would play hooky more; I would-n't make such good grades except by accident. I would ride on more merry-go-rounds – I'd pick more daisies!'

4. Identify your strategy or approach – learn and develop stress-control skills. The one constant factor in health care in the 21st century will be the need to accept and meet the challenge of change. By remaining flexible and accepting change as a challenge, we are more likely to respond to stress in a positive and healthy way. When we are flexible like a tall reed, we are able to sway against the winds of change – but when rigid we are much more liable to snap! Therefore, there is a need to learn and develop a flexible style of coping. List the stress-management options available to you and rate them in terms of their attractiveness. For example, decide how easy or difficult it will be to incor-porate an activity into your lifestyle. Does it appear to be comfortable or daunting; consider the risk of not sticking to a programme because failure can be a potential threat to one's self-esteem. Decide what out-come and result will be satisfactory and your chance of success or failure. In order to deal with a potential stress-inducing situation you might decide to:

a. do nothing – that is, the situation is likely to resolve itself without taking immediate action

b. compromise

c. learn to live with the situation

d. procrastinate or play for time; while this can be a negative stress-management technique, there are some occasions on which it might be useful and more beneficial than taking action (see the section on time management)

e. confront the situation or person

f. get someone else to handle the situation for you

g. learn and use certain skills such as:

    i. assertiveness – the capacity to influence or control other people without damaging the relationship; it is concerned with your point of view and views and interests of other people (Galassi et al. 1981) (see Chapter five on anger management)

    ii. relaxation (see the final chapter), meditation or yoga

    iii. venting steam (see the final chapter)

    iv. avoid faulty thinking – cognitive methods in the management of stress (refer to the final chapter)

    v. use an appropriate style of leadership

    vi. develop interpersonal and social skills – the job of the doctor involves dealing with other people as patients, colleagues and staff; socially unskilled doctors create high levels of discontent, job dissatisfaction and grievance for all concerned; the consequences of this for doctors, their colleagues and staff leads to loss of motivation, labour turnover and absenteeism – actual illness and sickness, or simply 'sick of work'

    vii. build and develop social support networks (see the final chapter)

    viii. conflict management (see Chapter five)

    viv. anger management (see Chapter five)

    x. time management, for example, speed-reading, effective writing techniques, the management of meetings (see Chapter three)

     xi. manage your Type A style of behaviour (see Chapter six)

    xii. role negotiation (see Chapter five) on anger management.

As we have noted, some of these techniques have already been discussed in Part Three of this book, 'Behaviour and stress', while others are described in detail in the final chapter.

5. Plan your activities – share and discuss your plan with another person or your immediate group. Draw up a timetable of your regular activities. This should be used as your implementation plan and must specifically state how you intend to achieve your aims and goals. You are more likely to stay committed to a plan of action if you share your ideas and goals with other people. Making a declaration will help you to stick to your objective. Ideally, use another person as a 'buddy' and ask them to check on your progress at regular intervals. If you reciprocate by acting as a buddy for a colleague you will develop a bond that will strengthen goal commitment and the likelihood of success.

6. Evaluate progress – reward success. Regularly evaluate, monitor and assess your actions by critically analyzing your progress and, if necessary, reformulating your plan. This will be easier to do if you have kept a written log. Also, your 'buddy' can help you to be objective in this assessment. Identify a worthy reward for actively and positively dealing with stress. Make sure you enjoy your promised reward. It is sometimes difficult for us to persist and work towards a distant goal because the likelihood of reaching the goal and the reward seems too remote. Overcome this problem by setting interim targets that will progressively move you towards your optimal goal. Ensure that you reward yourself for success at each target stage and on the achievement of your final goal.

7. Understand your preferred coping style. When faced with demand that we are unable to meet we will experience stress. At this time we resort to tried and tested

ways of coping that have helped us to deal with similar situations in the past. However, it is important to reassess the effectiveness of these strategies because we can develop ways of coping that cause harm or aggravate the problem. The issue of 'maladaptive behaviour' in response to stress has already been discussed. However, the examples in Table 7.1 serve as a reminder and illustrate the differences between adaptive and maladaptive styles of coping with stress. Use 'adaptive'

Table 7.1   Adaptive and maladaptive stress-coping styles

Stressor agent	Adaptive coping style	Maladaptive coping style
A serious disagreement with a doctor colleague concerning a patient Atmosphere very acrimonious and tense	Discuss the situation with your colleague in an overt, assertive way Negotiate and agree a solution	Attack your colleague through a third party and involve administrative staff by attempting to gain support and favour Argue with your colleague in public or in front of other colleagues
Far too much work to do in addition to the patient workload – not likely that you will meet the deadlines set	Delegate some work Ask a colleague to help in exchange for doing something for them at a later date Honour the agreement	Struggle to meet the demand with result that your general performance deteriorates – you become irritable with colleagues and at home Failure to meet deadline is compounded by a loss of self-esteem and confidence
You feel unable to keep up with the amount of professional reading required in order to remain informed about recent medical guidelines and procedures	Learn to speed-read Liase with colleagues to share the material and brief each other during a lunchtime meeting Make sure you have something to read when you have a few spare moments while waiting for your next meeting/appointment	Try and stay wake at night to read – fall asleep while reading in bed Continue to look at the growing pile of documents on your desk in despair Eventually throw half away without reading them

Table 7.1 *continued*

Relatives of a patient are continually demanding and difficult They insist in turning up at the surgery demanding to be seen and create an unsettling atmosphere for the practice reception staff	Discuss the situation with a colleague to obtain another perspective Ask the colleague to join you in a meeting with the people concerned Ensure the reception staff are trained to deal with the situation and that they have your support in this matter	Make sure that their phone calls are never put through to you Ignore their threats about taking the matter further Remain distant, and non-communicative when confronted
Feeling that your work and home life demands are seriously out of balance – not able to spend enough time with the family	Keep a time log of activities; examine time wasters; identify and create free-time periods and schedule in family and social activities Stick to your schedule and the plan	Ignore the complaints of family – work is more important Anyway, you have a 10-day holiday planned 5 months from now – they should be grateful that you are taking them to the Maldives!

coping strategies – avoid maladaptive coping; do not let stress control you, learn to exert control.

8. Maintain positive interactions with other people. Give other people as much responsibility as they can handle. Say thank you for the efforts of others and remember that praise is one of the most powerful ways to reinforce desired behaviour. Know when to 'push' others and when not to. Accept and give social support to the people around you. Ask yourself, 'Are you a stress carrier?' Some people are just like 'typhoid Mary'; they do not suffer from the affects of the disease themselves, but infect everyone around them. Are you, without realizing it, creating stress for your colleagues, family or friends? Can you change?

9. Stay fit, healthy and happy to cope with stress that is an inevitable part of working and living as a medical practitioner. Maintain a healthy and balanced lifestyle – good nutrition, diet and health are often controversial topics, and changing advice creates confusion and

misunderstanding. However, a balanced diet, 'moderation in all things', the avoidance of drug and substance abuse, and good sleep habits, all help to keep us fit to cope with stress. Stay physically activity by taking regular, moderate exercise (see the final chapter). Use humour – smile and the world will smile with you; weep and you weep alone. The desire to please seems to be a natural emotion and so people tend to smile back in response to a smile. Other people are more likely to relax in your presence and be less difficult if they are greeted with a smile. If you are angry or upset, try 'thought-stopping' and then use mental diversion (see final chapter) by thinking about a positive and amusing experience. It is impossible to stay angry and keep a smile on your face. Smile when you are talking on the telephone. It will help to make you sound more friendly, approachable and positive. As we have said before, aggression breeds aggression. Use signs and posters in the work place to encourage smiles. Start the day with your favourite, amusing 'thought or joke for the day' calendar.

10. Get professional help and seek social support. It is sometimes difficult for the medical practitioner, as a carer of other people, to admit that they cannot cope, or need help. Other people have stress . . . . not the doctor! Also, we seem to inhabit a world where superman and superwoman reign supreme and, of course, we tend to aspire to follow these role models. Stress is perceived as a 'four-letter-word', because it equates to the inability to cope with one's job, or life – stress, in these terms is failure and non-coping. Until we accept that stress is inevitable and that we are not superhuman, but potentially vulnerable, it is unlikely that we will effectively control stress. Although we advocate that the elimination of a source of stress is the most effective approach to the management of strain and pressure, it is realistic to acknowledge that this advice is not always practical for doctors. Busy doctors are well intentioned and during stress-management

seminars will write positive action plans with the vow to take more exercise, learn to relax and drink less alcohol. However, it is well known that the road to hell is paved with good intentions, and so doctors, just like their patients, will become casualties of stress. At this point the need to seek and use professional help and support is essential. If the findings reported by Graham et al. (2001) are representative of doctors in general, we can assume that this is not a coping option that the medical practitioner will readily use or admit to using (see section on maladaptive coping). Therefore, the following strategies are suggested:

a. Ask for help – sometimes our attempts to cope with stress are ineffective and we become a victim of stress. At these times it is important to ask for help as soon as possible. However, to do this, we need to be able to recognize the signs and symptoms of stress in ourselves and other people (refer to Chapter one). Sometimes we cannot see a problem developing until it is too late. Indeed, stress trends to creep up in an insidious manner and so having a 'buddy' at work, who is able to recognize our negative reactions to the strain and pressures of work life, and help by gently moving us away from harm (physically and emotionally), is an important asset.

b. Use social support – having a supportive culture and climate at work and at home will ensure that there are people around us who will try to help. Remember to give and accept social support. However, there are times when we may not be able to turn to colleagues and family for support. At these times the help of trained professionals who can offer counselling to deal with stress-related problems should be considered (see the final chapter for guidance on social support stress coping strategies).

c. Use a counselling service – according to the British Association of Counselling's (BAC) Code for Counsellors, the overall aim of counselling is to provide an opportunity for a client to work towards living in a more satisfied and resourceful way. They also state that counselling may be concerned with developmental issues, addressing and resolving specific problems, making decisions, coping with crisis, developing personal insight and knowledge, working through feelings of inner conflict or improving relationships with others. Further, the counsellor's role is to facilitate the client's work in ways which respect the client's values, personal resources and capacity for self-determination (BAC 1992). Thus the aim is to increase the individual's capacity to withstand a perceived stressor. Counselling is often described as a conversation with the purpose of providing a client with an opportunity to explore, discover and clarify ways of living more resourcefully and towards a greater well-being.

According to Pereira Gray (1988) it has been estimated that as many as one-third of all patients who consult a doctor do so because they have a personal problem or real physical symptoms causing them distress but reflecting an underlying psychosocial problem. It is suggested that doctors might not recognize the potential benefits of counselling, but may medicalize 'life-problems' or psychosomatic symptoms because they lack psychological training. Likewise, doctors may not appreciate the benefits of counselling for their own similar problems.

According to Allen and Bor (1997) the psychological benefits of counselling, the presence of a counsellor in the primary healthcare team leads to a reduction in patients' psychosomatic symptoms, a consequent reduction in drug prescription rates, and a reduction in the demand for the time of medical staff. Other claimed benefits include fewer inappropriate referrals and investigations, and fewer hospital admissions, thus reducing the workload of the doctor. It appears that the division of workload leads to increased satisfaction for GPs and greater mutual respect within the primary healthcare team (Allen & Bor 1997). Some doctors have also adopted many of the skills used in the counselling context, such as active listening, empathetic responding and reflection, as part of the move towards a 'patient-centred' approach to medical care. Both the doctor and the patient benefit from the improvement in communication and the subsequent increased patient and professional satisfaction, greater diagnostic adequacy, and improved adherence to treatment (Davis & Fallowfield 1991). This is very important since poor communication accounts for some of the reasons given by patients for unsatisfactory medical consultations (Ley 1988) and this is cited as central to the reasons why patients sue their professional carers (Beckman et al. 1994).

Cooper et al. (1992) have shown how the provision of a counselling service at work can significantly reduce the amount of time lost through sickness absence and improve self-reported psychological health. Psychological counselling services are now available to patients in many practice surgeries, and offered by health authorities for use by doctors, but resistance to counselling still exists. This problem is common in many public and private sector organizations. The workforce remains concerned about using counselling to deal with stress-related problems because they fear the stigma of using psychological therapy (Sibicky & Dovidio 1986) and the subsequent label of 'non-coper'. Thus, the need for confidentiality is paramount. West and Reynolds (1995) suggest that attitudes to, and take up of counselling services within organizational settings can be improved by:

i. clearly demonstrating confidentiality

ii. showing that people who seek counselling are actively and positively taking care of themselves and displaying an effective reaction to stress. This counteracts the traditional picture of the helpless dependant seeking counselling (Sibicky & Dovidio 1986)

      iii. a positive management attitude to counselling and use of the service.

d. Use an employee assistance programme – external counselling can take the form of a service which is described as an employee assistance programme (EAP). A company contracts an EAP provider to give employees, and sometimes their immediate families, access to an independent, confidential advice and short-term counselling service. In addition to work-related problems, relationship difficulties, illness worries, redundancy or retirement concerns, substance abuse, or financial worries might be presented and dealt with by the EAP provider. First contact with the EAP provider is by telephone, and can be on a referral or self-referral basis. If necessary, meetings are arranged off-site at professional consulting rooms. Research evidence suggests that EAP counselling-based interventions seem to have a positive impact in terms of:

      i.   improved psychological health – less anxiety and depression

      ii. feeling better and more able to cope

      iii. the resolution of a problem

      iv. many users have said that they would use an EAP again

      v. improved self-esteem

      vi. a tendency to engage in more adaptive stress-coping behaviours, such as yoga or exercise

      vii. a decrease in sickness absences.

One of the main criticisms of counselling as a stress-management technique is that it treats symptoms rather than tackling the stress agent. This criticism is acknowledged, and the EAP providers now attempt to feed back this type of information to the organization. For example, if the cause of a problem is identified as the inconsiderate and bullying doctor, simply providing counselling to the distressed and depressed employee, who habitually stays away from work to avoid the boss, will not resolve this issue. After counselling, this member of staff is likely to feel better and more able to cope, but still has to face the difficult doctor. Thus, the management style of the doctor should be examined, and if necessary, re-training offered to deal with the problem.

11. Stay in control – life is stress – don't less stress control you! It is important that we feel in control of pressure and stress in life. Karasek and Theorell (1990) have described the importance of control as a buffer against the strains and pressures associated with a high demand job. It seems that we are more likely to cope with the pressure of a demanding job if we also feel in control of the things that affect us at work. Having autonomy in the job means being consulted and taking part in the decisions that affect you and the way in which you do the job. Figure 7.1 illustrates the job demand–control model proposed by Karasek and Theorell, which states that we can understand response to job demands if we also take into account the person's perception of 'control' in the workplace. Thus, the combined effects of a high demand with low job control (that is, a lack of opportunity to make decisions or have a say about the way the job is done)

Job demands – control – social support and response to stress

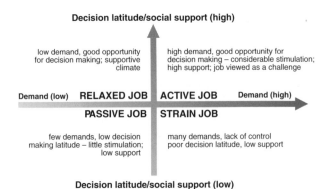

Figure 7.1   Job demands – control – social support and the stress response

creates negative emotions and associated physiological stress reactions, which in the long term can adversely affect health and well-being. This type of job is described as a 'strain' job, compared to the 'active' job that is also very demanding, but offers discretion and autonomy.

It is suggested that the job of medical practitioner has become a 'strain' occupation because certain aspects of job control have been taken away. Doctors no longer have such a high level of discretion as in the past because clinical autonomy is diminished. Indeed, the imposition of the 1990 GP contract by the UK government was viewed as an attack on the 'independent' contractor status and professional autonomy of GPs (Calnan & Williams 1995, Lewis 1997), and doctors in Canada and the USA have been the recipients of similar action. Nevertheless, it is important for medical practitioners to find ways of gaining control and the perception of being 'in-control', rather than 'controlled', in order to minimize the damaging consequences of exposure to a demanding job.

12. Stress is a dynamic process. The management of stress should become an on-going process, not a one-off course, session or stress-management programme. Attendance at a stress-management seminar will only be beneficial if it leads to action and change at the end of the day – not if the experience simply means another shiny manual on the bookshelf! Therefore, it is important to integrate stress control activities into the day-to-day work life of the doctor, the general practice, or the hospital department or ward.

To be successful, stress management must be the joint responsibility of every doctor and every employer in medical practice. This means that an employer has a duty of care towards the employee to ensure that they are not damaged physically or psychologically by the nature of the job. Also, each member of staff has a duty of care to ensure that they remain fit and able to do the job, as contracted, without causing harm to themselves or other people at work. This means, that whenever possible, strategies to prevent stress problems from arising should be considered. As Kompier and Levi (1994) suggest:

a. eliminating or modifying the stress-producing situation or removing the doctor from it; find 'the right shoe for the right foot', or allow the doctor concerned to adjust the 'shoe' to fit the foot

b. adjusting the 'shoe' – that is, change the work to fit the doctor's foot

c. strengthening the doctor's resilience to stress, for example, through physical exercise, meditation, relaxation or social support; this includes training to alter the person's response to stress, and to ensure that the response is positive rather than harmful.

In the final chapter we provide details of some of the options for the management and control of stress and explain why we emphasize the importance of self-management as an effective stress-management strategy for doctors.

chapter EIGHT

Stress control strategies

The competing demands on time and the steadily increasing volume of work continue to cause worrying levels of stress and burnout among doctors. In the conclusion of a recent review of research conducted by the British Medical Association (Beecham 2000) of senior hospital doctors and GPs, they suggested that the remedies for this problem were straightforward and recommended:

1. increasing the number of consultants
2. the evaluation of work demands and the review of staffing
3. implementing the working time directive that caps hours at 48 per week
4. introducing more flexible employment practices
5. encouraging uptake of annual leave and study leave
6. organizing properly trained locum cover (Beecham 2000).

Whilst we support these recommendations completely, and suspect that many similar surveys have recognized the need to take such action to alleviate the problem of stress and burnout among doctors, we contend that doctors need to take action at a personal and individual level to self-manage the stress of working in medical practice. Many of the initiatives described above take time to put in place and become effective, and others, sadly, will remain part of a well-intentioned but idealistic goal. Indeed, the same study found that doctors complain that they have little control over their workload and lack adequate resources for the job. Also, a key source of stress was the sharing of emotional distress and physical suffering of the patients. In such circumstances many of the options usually recommended as part of a stress-prevention programme are not viable or timely. In short, we believe that doctors need to accept that the maxim, 'physician heal thyself' (Luke iv. 23) must be reinterpreted as, 'physician – take care of thyself'. Therefore, this final chapter provides details of self-management stress-control strategies. These include:

- relaxation techniques and breathing exercises
- venting steam
- cognitive methods in the management of stress
- the role of social support in stress management
- exercise and stress control
- career breaks – that is, 'getting off the hot seat'.

Relaxation

We have acknowledged that Type A doctors find it difficult to relax and tend to feel guilty when not working. However, learning to relax is an important stress-management skill for all doctors. Relaxation training, meditation or yoga can be used to reduce levels of arousal and moderate the stress response. One of the active ingredients in the deleterious impact of psychological stress on physical health might be its role in depleting levels of secretory immunoglobin-A (S-IgA). This is the first line of defence against infections such as colds and coughs. Acute stress, for example, giving a short presentation, increases levels of S-IgA, but chronic stress results in lowered levels of S-IgA and subsequent increases in the frequencies of ill health (Wetherall 2002). Recent findings indicate that relaxation and massage might protect against illness because these stress ameliorators can increase levels of S-IgA (Bristow, cited in Wetherall 2002). Psychologically, successful relaxation results in enhanced feelings of well-being, peacefulness, a sense of personal control and a reduction in feelings of tension and anxiety. Therefore, the physiological benefits of relaxation include:

- a decrease in blood pressure
- slower respiration and heart rate
- reduced muscle tension
- less stomach acid
- lower levels of cholesterol
- alpha and theta brain waves to enhance creative and cognitive processes.

Relaxation techniques are simple to learn, but must be practised regularly if any benefits are to be gained. By learning and using controlled breathing and relaxation techniques, the doctor can reduce tension at will, and develop the ability to adapt to stressful situations at work or home. The first and essential skill in successful relaxation is correct breathing. Controlled breathing helps us to confront a source of stress, maintain self-control and decrease the emotional impact of the stressor. It acts at mechanical, chemical and nervous levels and aids muscle relaxation – this results in an immediate reduction of stress and emotional and mental tension. Relaxation allows the individual to discharge emotional tension that has built up in the body. The technique helps one to recover quickly from accumulated psychological and physical fatigue. In time, the doctor will develop a capacity not only to cope with, but also to resist stress.

Relaxation techniques

Relaxation techniques vary greatly and include autogenic training (Schultz & Luthe 1959); progressive, deep-muscle relaxation techniques (Jacobson 1929); meditation or simply a brief period of mental and physical relaxation while sitting comfortably in a chair in the workplace or at home. A wide variety of biofeedback devices, music therapy and audiotapes are available to guide and aid our ability to relax. These need to be chosen carefully because a spoken voice or music that is perceived to be irritating is not likely to aid the process of relaxation.

One helpful routine requires the individual to tense and relax muscle groups in turn and in a set order.

- Sit in a comfortable position in a chair that supports your back and neck, or lay down on the floor with your head supported by a cushion.
- Find a quiet, warm place where you will not be interrupted; close your eyes.
- Begin by taking in a few deep breaths through the nose, and exhaling to push the air out of the lungs through the mouth.
- Continue to breath deeply and slowly, while tensing groups of muscles for 10 seconds, and then relaxing each group for 30 seconds – using the following order:

    1. clench fists and relax
    2. bend arms to flex the biceps and then straighten
    3. straighten arms tightly to flex the triceps – relax
    4. shrug shoulders up towards the ears and then drop them to relax
    5. press head back to tense the neck muscles and relax
    6. purse lips and relax
    7. press the tongue against back of teeth and relax
    8. clench teeth to tense the jaw and relax
    9. squeeze eyes tightly shut, frown and then relax
    10. breathe in deeply and hold to tense the chest – exhale deeply and relax
    11. tense the stomach muscles as if preparing them for a blow and relax
    12. clench the buttock muscles together tightly and relax
    13. keep legs straight without locking the knees – point the toes downwards and then relax.

- Make a commitment to PRACTICE EACH DAY for 1 month to assess the benefits.
- Remember this thirteen-point schedule and keep to the set routine – it becomes easier with time.
- Always end your relaxation session with several deep breaths. Then after slowly opening your eyes, maintain

your relaxation position for a few minutes before resuming your next activity.
• Play music to help you to relax.

It is possible to purchase a variety of tools that monitor the physiological reactions of the body to stress. This means it is possible to monitor the state of relaxation. For example, a commercially manufactured stress dot can be applied to a fleshy part of the hand between the base of the forefinger and thumb. This responds to skin temperature. When we are stressed or tense, the supply of blood is diverted away from the skin surface because it is needed to prepare the body for 'fight or flight'. As we relax, the blood supply will flow nearer to the skin surface for cooling purposes and the 'dot' will change colour to reflect this change. This provides a visual cue of the stress response and the process is known as 'biofeedback'. Other gadgets are available to monitor pulse or heart rate. However, it should be recognized that levels of sophistication, reliability and cost vary greatly, but such aids can assist in the process of understanding the physiological nature of stress.

Short relaxation exercises

Doctors tend to be constantly time-driven and so find it difficult to make a regular commitment to an exercise or relaxation routine that takes them away from work activity for a long period of time. Although the exercise described above should take only 20–25 minutes, the following routines are briefer and so might be beneficial at the start of a stress-management programme. The time-obsessed Type A doctor will find the approach particularly appealing because they take only 5–10 minutes to practise. The aim is to evoke feeling of peace and relaxation whenever desired.

A 5–10-minute relaxation session

• Select a comfortable sitting or reclining position.
• Close your eyes and think about a place that you have been before that represents your ideal place for physical

and mental relaxation. It should be a quiet environment, perhaps the seashore, the mountains or even your own back garden. If you can't think of an ideal relaxation place, then create one in your mind.

- Now imagine that you are actually in your ideal relaxation place. Imagine that you are seeing all the colours, hearing the sounds, and able to taste and smell the aromas. Just lie back, and enjoy your soothing, rejuvenating environment.
- Feel the peacefulness, the calmness, and imagine your whole body and mind being renewed and refreshed.
- After 5–10 minutes, slowly open your eyes and stretch. You have the realization that you may instantly return to your relaxation place whenever you desire, and experience a peacefulness and calmness in body and mind.

Momentary relaxation

The relaxation exercises described above require an investment in time, but when you have learned to achieve a state of deep relaxation you can also begin to draw upon your memory of relaxation to achieve partial relaxation during the day. Taking a few deep, slow breaths can often bring on this feeling of relaxation. Albrecht (1979) states that the skill of momentary relaxation should come almost automatically once an individual has mastered a deep-relaxation technique. With the following examples he describes the feeling of momentary relaxation:

- The next time you find yourself about to deal with a challenging, stressful situation, simply pause for a few seconds, turn your attention to your body and allow your whole body to relax as much as you can, keeping the situation in mind. You can easily learn to do this 'quickie' relaxation technique in a few seconds and without the slightest outward sign of what you are doing. Anyone looking at you would notice, at most, that you had become silent and that you seemed to be thinking about something for a few seconds. You need not even close your eyes to do this.

- If you happen to have a few moments alone before entering a challenging situation, you can relax yourself somewhat more thoroughly. Sit down, if possible, get comfortable and close your eyes. Use your built-in muscle memory to bring back the feeling of deep relaxation and hold it for about a full minute. Then open your eyes and, as you go about the task at hand, try to retain the feeling of calmness that came with the relaxation.

Other techniques including meditation, self-hypnosis, biofeedback and autogenic training may be used in order to relax. These usually require the help of experts and/or therapists and require training over a period of time to induce a general feeling of well-being and high-stress coping ability.

A breathing exercise

Until people begin to learn and practice relaxation techniques they are usually not aware that they have developed poor breathing habits. Part of the relaxation process is the ability to breathe deeply and slowly. During the process of relaxation it is suggested that we breathe in as deeply as possible through the nose, momentarily hold this air in our lungs, and then exhale by pushing the air out through the mouth and making a 'whooshing' sound. It is also possible to improve your breathing by strengthening the diaphragm. If you are a singer or a public speaker you have probably been trained to do this already. It is known as 'bellows breathing' and it improves the blood oxygenation process. When you have learned the technique below, use bellows breathing twice a day to give an oxygen rush to the brain. You can do this on waking, before an important and potentially stressful work activity, or to overcome the after-lunch 'dip' or late afternoon 'slump'. The rush of oxygen will wake up the brain and you will feel re-charged. Whilst we cannot say that you will be able to sing like The Great Caruso, the tone and quality of your voice will improve if your regularly practice bellows breathing.

Bellows breathing

- Place your hands across your torso – the palms over the lower part of the ribcage. Your fingertips should meet just below your sternum. This is the diaphragm and you should be able to feel it moving as you breathe.
- Using this muscle, fill your lungs. Concentrate on pushing your diaphragm out against the slight resistance from your fingers. If you are doing this correctly the mouth and lungs will take in air.
- Using the diaphragm alone, breathe in and out rapidly. Almost as if you are panting.
- Make sure that your shoulders are not rising and falling and your chest should not expand much.
- Allow the diaphragm to draw quick, shallow breaths for 30 seconds or more, up to a minute, but stop if you start to feel dizzy. With practice you will able to improve on your initial performance.

The body needs time to relax and recuperate from the effects of everyday strains and pressures. Some doctors can dissipate stress easily whiles others appear to bury it deep inside. For these people life seems to be a series of crises. The chronically uptight individual tends to meet even minor problems as if they are critical incidents. A disagreement with a colleague, a difficult consultation with a patient, a delay in the delivery of new equipment, or problems with a teenage son or daughter, all take on the same apparent magnitude for the uptight doctor who is unable to relax. Such a person meets the smallest problem situation with an unnecessarily intense reaction (Albrecht 1979). Learning to relax can help to mitigate the physical response to stress and aid the coping process. However, some situations might be confronted in a more positive way if the individual is allowed to 'vent steam' as part of the stress-coping process. This is discussed next.

Venting steam

Often a stressful experience will become more difficult to deal with because we need to bottle-up the symptoms. Typically, doctors are not able to overtly express true feelings and emotions in the work environment whilst dealing with patients. Also, those doctors who tend to be aggressive and exhibit the Type A style of behaviour usually internalize their emotions. Although some doctors will discharge their wrath and aggression towards other people in the work environment, it is more likely that they continue to rage inside because it is inappropriate to express aggression or anger overtly. The Type A individual also tends to seethe inside as self-imposed deadlines and goals are not realized, or feelings of frustration arise because of dissatisfaction with the efforts of colleagues and staff.

Some guidance on anger and conflict management has been suggested already in Chapter five. However, it is also possible to dissipate stress and find relief by 'venting steam'. Simply talking about a situation or writing about strong feelings might be helpful because the stress situation is externalized rather than bottled-up inside. Venting frustration and anger to an understanding colleague, friend or member of the family is one of the most common ways of venting steam. The practice of writing down your feelings can also reduce the emotions associated with conflict or anger. It is the reason why we suggest this process as part of the daily stress-log process (see Appendix I). Keeping a regular journal of your feelings allows you to reflect back and identify any common themes or patterns associated with these negative and potentially damaging emotions. Even having an animated and loud discussion with yourself while driving and spending time in the car alone can be a way of venting steam

You might prefer to vent steam by writing that angry letter. We suggest that you do not send it, but keep it somewhere safe, and read it later when you feel calm and in control. At this point you can revise and send it, or simply tear it up in to many pieces – also a therapeutic exercise! Some people prefer to vent steam through the process of vigorous and physical activity. Anger can be released by imagining the face of a difficult colleague, patient or other antagonist on a golf, cricket or squash ball as it is hit firmly and hard! We have suggested that 'having a conversation with one's self' can be a form of venting steam, however, the existence of certain faulty thought processes can create chronic stress. Therefore in the next section we consider the role of cognition in the stress management process.

Cognitive methods in the management of stress

Cognitive distortions can arise in response to stressful events and cognitive behaviour therapy was developed from the acknowledged relationship between maladaptive thinking and anxiety and stress (Beck et al. 1985). This assumes that negative, irrational thought patterns will distort the perception and evaluation of a threatening stimulus and thus prevent adaptive coping-oriented behaviour (Bruch 1997). Cognitive techniques are used to raise awareness of cognitive distortion that exists as irrational, negative and dysfunctional thoughts. Therefore, we can reduce or eliminate a potentially stressful situation by learning to perceive stress differently by avoiding faulty thinking. The way in which a doctor perceives a situation will determine the stress-response outcome. For example, doctors who exhibit Type A coronary-prone patterns of behaviour continually activate the stress response by perceiving life as highly competitive and time driven, often because they set unrealistic and unachievable goals for themselves and the people who work with them. Cognitive reappraisal of such situations can be used to avoid negative and harmful outcomes.

Cognitive coping strategies

Occupational stress is perceived as a transactional process whereby a doctor will appraise a situation and react to a potential source of stress. Cognitive style influences this process and the coping strategy subsequently used. Research evidence suggests that the use of certain coping strategies, such as avoidance, are associated with poor psychological well-being, whilst the use of problem-oriented coping is linked to positive mental health (Guppy & Weatherstone 1997). Further, Beck (1987) suggests that individuals are instrumental in creating their own negative feelings by having irrational beliefs and that dysfunctional attitudes produce clinical symptomology. For example:

- Vulnerability, such as, 'Whenever I take a chance or risk, I am only looking for trouble' or 'People will reject you if they know your weaknesses'
- Need for approval, such as, 'I need other people's approval for me to be happy'
- Success-perfectionism, such as, 'My life is wasted unless I am a success' and 'I must be a useful, productive or creative person or life has no meaning'
- Imperatives, such as,' I should be happy all the time' 'I should always have complete control over my feelings' and 'I should try to impress other people if I want them to like me'.

The use of cognitive restructuring as a stress-management technique aims to examine dysfunctional attitudes and irrational thoughts. The objective is to improve the balance between the perception of a demand and the ability to cope with that demand. It involves thinking about stressful events to make them seem less threatening by challenging irrational beliefs. Thus, reactions to a situation are changed by the way in which the circumstances are perceived. A variety of techniques are available to help in the cognitive re-appraisal of stressful situations. The individual is encouraged to examine beliefs, thoughts, feelings, actions and the consequences of these, in order to identify rational versus irrational beliefs. A rational belief is one that sits comfortably with you and your outlook on life, whilst an irrational belief is one that causes discomfort or distress. We tend to hold distorted or irrational beliefs in a variety of ways.

- Jumping to conclusions – this error is described as 'selective abstraction' and involves concentrating on some detail taken out of context, while ignoring more conspicuous features of the event. Thus, we jump to a conclusion when there is no appropriate evidence or fact to justify this assumption. For example, we conclude that someone dislikes us because they fail to turn up for a meeting, when in reality other reasons, such as the current public transport strike, could more accurately explain this situation.
- Selective perception – this usually happens when we try to justify our own unacceptable behaviour by refusing to consider the reality of the situation. For example, 'I had to drive even though I had had too much to drink . . . . It was an emergency'.
- Ignore important details – this is also known as minimization and involves focusing on one detail taken out of its context and ignoring more important aspects of the event. For example, feeling hopeless and a failure because you did not get a promotion, but ignoring the fact that six other doctors on the promotion board were turned down also and many others did not even reach the short list.
- Overgeneralization – means drawing some general rule or conclusions from one or a few isolated events and assuming that it can be applied to all similar or dissimilar circumstances. For example, assuming that you are hopeless at everything you do, and punishing yourself excessively and repeatedly because you found one mistake on a twenty-page review paper; or, 'My colleague was attacked on XYZ Street; I will be attacked when I visit my patient living in that district'.
- Exaggerate the importance of things – also known as magnification. This type of distortion occurs when we think that a situation is vital or very significant, when in reality it is trivial. For example, automatically assum-

ing that something awful is about to happen because you have been asked to go to a meeting that you are not usually invited to attend.

• Take things personally – this type of cognitive distortion is known as personalization and refers to the individual's proclivity to believe that things happening around us, especially negative ones, are somehow related to us in an important way, even when there is no rationale for this. For example, the senior consultant asks everyone to take extra care with the preparations for an imminent VIP visit and inspection. You assume that this is a criticism directed to you alone, even though the request was presented to everyone at an open meeting – the director was 'getting at you'.

• Black and white thinking – also known as dichotomous or 'all or none thinking'. This means that we tend to see things only in terms of one or two categories – usually extreme dichotomies, without room for anything in between these viewpoints. Usually the individual adopts the most negative classification.

To avoid falling into such traps it is necessary to examine thoughts and feelings in order to detect and define misattributions. A five-step approach is recommended for refuting irrational ideas:

1. Write down the facts – detect the irrationality.
2. Write down your thoughts and feelings – debate against the irrationalities.
3. Focus on your emotional response.
4. Dispute and change the irrational thought or notion – discriminate between rational and irrational thought:
   a. Is there any support for the idea?
   b. What is the evidence for the falseness of the idea?
   c. Does any evidence exist for the truth of the idea?
   d. What is the worst thing that could happen?
   e. What good things might occur if . . . . ?
5. Substitute alternate patterns of thought – maintain close contact with reality.

It is also suggested that we engage in a mental monologue and convert destructive self-talk into constructive self-talk.

Mental monologue

Flexibility in thinking about a situation is necessary in order to manage stress effectively. By taking a problem-solving approach and re-appraising the situation in a rational way we avoid stress-inducing situations. The following four-step approach is recommended in order to retain positive thoughts:

1. Constructive self-talk. Quick and Quick (1984) described the process of 'constructive self-talk'. Self-talk is an 'intermittent mental monologue' that most people conduct about the events they experience and their reactions to these events. This monologue or self-talk can range from being gently positive to harshly condemning. When someone engages in negative self-talk they achieve nothing, sustain the stress response, and place demands upon their physical and emotional energy reserves. Therefore, it is suggested that constructive self-talk can be used as an effective stress-control strategy. By focussing on the positive aspects of a situation, holding realistic expectations, and keeping things in perspective, it is possible to avoid damage caused by negative thoughts. Quick and Quick have provided examples of constructive self-talk. Ultimately their advice is to avoid negative, destructive thoughts that create a vicious downward spiral of stress. For example, anticipation of an opportunity to present a conference paper or research results will become destructive if the typical mental monologue is:

What if I make a mistake; what if people can't hear me because I talk too fast or mumble when I am nervous; what if they ask questions I cannot answer? I hate public speaking; why did I agree to do it?

Obsessive worry can only drain your emotional resources, leading to disaster, and the likelihood of avoidance of public speaking in the future. Compare this to a constructive self-talk monologue:

This will be a challenge. I have a prompt card to remind me to breathe correctly so I don't mumble or speak too quickly. It is a good piece of research. They will be interested and enjoy it. I have rehearsed, so I know my stuff. If someone asks a question and I do not know the answer I will say so, and offer to find out and let him/her know soon. I cannot be expected to know everything.

2. Quick recovery. It is also important to combine a monologue process with the technique of 'quick recovery'. This is the ability to bounce back from an upsetting experience. We sometimes prolong or exacerbate a negative experience because we continually re-visit it in our mind to try and justify our position or rehash the event. It is just like using a video replay to return to the scene, but instead of doing this to learn from the experience, and then move on, we get caught up in a continuous loop that becomes more and more punishing and damaging with each re-play. The 'quick recovery' approach suggests that you stop this negative and damaging circular loop by becoming more rational and less conscious of the need to win on every occasion. Quick and Quick suggest that we can avoid damage by using the techniques of 'thought stopping' and 'mental diversion'.

3. Thought stopping. 'Thought stopping' means recognizing non-constructive thoughts, attitudes and behaviours, and stopping them immediately by visualizing, for example, a large 'STOP' traffic sign. One doctor explained that he used this technique to switch off thoughts of work on arrival home by looking at a large, red stop sign placed on the wall immediately opposite the door.

4. Mental diversion. After using the 'thought stopping' process use 'mental diversion' to divert your thoughts to a topic that is more comfortable and manageable, or

until you are ready to cope with the stress event. Diverting one's thoughts to a more pleasant and restful subject can stop a negative train of thought and subsequent drain on energy reserves. It should not be confused with 'denial' as a coping mechanism because this tactic can be harmful.

Although we suggest that a mental monologue can help to avoid faulty thinking and dissipate irrational beliefs, the ability to discuss our thoughts, hopes and fears with a considerate and empathetic colleague, spouse, or friend is highly recommended as a method of managing a potentially stressful situation. The role of social support in the management of stress is discussed in the next section.

The role of social support in stress management

The time-driven, workaholic style of behaviour of many doctors, in particular the Type A individual, often ignores the value of developing good social relationships at work. However, the value of social support as a buffer against the effects of strain and pressure is well documented. For example, Sutherland and Cooper (1992) found that social support was strongly linked to both job satisfaction and levels of depression among GPs, particularly the male respondents, who did not appear to use social support as a coping strategy in the same way as the female GPs in this study. Therefore, the value of emotional support in one's social network as a protection against adverse environmental forces or negative life events should not be underestimated. Whilst research evidence suggests that gender differences exist, and different sources of support appear to buffer the impact of different sources of stress, there is much evidence to suggest that social support can play a significant role in enhancing the level of well-being among medical practitioners and support staff. Doctors should actively encourage a more supportive work climate and ensure that social support networks involving both family and social interactions are well developed. As we have said, the doctor with a Type A style of behaviour often does not appreciate the importance of the role of social support as a stress-coping strategy. Social support as a stress-management strategy could be developed or improved in the following ways:

- It is necessary to emphasize the importance of supportive relationships and networks during the selection, recruitment and training of doctors in order to promote a supportive climate and culture. The culture of an organization affects the quality of working relationships, and so a supportive image needs to be encouraged, reinforced and acknowledged.
- Social support from the boss seems to be a very important source of support in the perception and mediation of job strain (refer to figure 7.1 on page 142). It has both a direct main effect and a buffering effect, and lack of support from one's boss is associated with perceived job strain, job dissatisfaction, and poor physical and psychological health. Therefore, it is necessary that doctors as managers of other people are trained to understand this need and reflect it in their style of management and supervision. It is also very important that each doctor is able to develop and maintain a supportive relationship with an immediate supervisor. This can be very important at the beginning of a career in medicine. For example, junior doctors cite 'difficult relationships with senior doctors' as a key source of stress (Firth-Cozens 1993). Also, Paice et al. (1997) found that satisfaction with the post was directly related to the amount of time consultants dedicated to supervision and training, including feedback and appraisal of junior doctors. Indeed, it must be acknowledged that membership of a well-functioning team can decrease stress levels and increase performance (Sonnetag 1996).
- Coherent teamwork is crucial for the delivery of good-quality patient care both directly in terms of efficient and effective services, and indirectly via its impact on stress reduction (Firth-Cozens 1998). In addition to the

opportunities for support and supervision, effective multidisciplinary teams can facilitate a review of the context of patient care and the resulting innovative work-patterns can minimize sleep deprivation (Read et al. 1988). For example, McKee and Black (1993) suggest that collaboration between managers, doctors, nurses and other professions would enable many of the tasks and questions about patient care at night to be carried out by staff other than doctors. Further, Firth-Cozens states that:

Rotas and on-call commitments need to be organised in the context of the daily activity of the team. Outpatient clinics, endoscopy lists, and routine surgery need not be scheduled to coincide with a team's responsibilities for medical care. And on-call commitments for emergencies should be understood as a 48-hour commitment – the day of and the day of 'take'. Moreover, work patterns may need to respond to the experience – or inexperience of team members. Do consultants, for example, reduce their or their registrars' clinic lists in order to support the new pre-registration house officers in that first week of August?

The message is clear – multi-professional clinical teams can only exist to offer effective healthcare and social support for medical professionals in a culture where good organizational practice is the norm.

- In addition to the use of clinical teams, the development of structures to provide more social support, including occupational health services, counselling programmes and employee assistance programmes are recommended as part of a stress-management programme.
- The development of social networks, both work and socially orientated, and self-help groups (for example, the use of 'health circles') should be encouraged in the practice surgery, clinic or hospital ward or department.
- Education about the importance of social support between work and home life is necessary so that doctors, and the spouse or partner of doctors understand

the value of social support, and the damaging consequences of lack of supportive relationships at home.

- The development of social support networks plays a significant part in enhancing the level of employee well-being, particularly social support from a boss. Self-managed work teams, or action groups all play a part in the development of social support networks, particularly for individuals who work in relative isolation. However, doctors working in general practice usually work within a group practice with a senior partner, and they tend to report feeling isolated because of the limited opportunity to meet and socialize with their colleagues. Likewise, the opportunity to meet with colleagues can be restricted for overloaded hospital doctors. To overcome this problem and develop a more supportive work culture, it is necessary to find time for both work and social gatherings for those in the group-practice surgery. Likewise, self-help groups or action groups in a hospital setting will achieve the same aims. Social support helps to moderate the stress–strain relationship by creating a feeling of belonging and solidarity, and it can have a positive effect on mood. It is also suggested that a lack of strong bonding, compounded by feelings of isolation, leads people to engage in non-compliant behaviours. These include absenteeism, tardiness, putting in less effort at work, and engaging in idle gossip, and so on, particularly when job security is threatened (Lim 1997).

There are a number of steps a doctor can take to find social support at work:

- Choose someone you feel you can talk to. This should be a person you do not feel threatened by and to whom you can reveal your feelings with trust. Be careful not to use others as pawns in the game of medical politics.
- Approach this person and explain that you have a particular problem at work (or outside of work), which you would like to discuss. Admit that you need help and that you think the person is the best person to consult

because you trust their views and opinion, and feel that they can identify with your circumstances.

- Try to build and maintain this relationship even at times when there is no crisis or problem.
- Continue to review the relationship to see if it is still providing you with the emotional support you need to cope with difficulties that arise. If the nature of the relationship changes you will need to seek help from a new direction.
- Co-counselling is a useful exercise to help both parties in a mutual support relationship. Another way of developing supportive relationships is to encourage a 'buddy' system so that you engage in social activities with another doctor rather than alone. Taking exercise in a group is usually an effective way of adhering to a programme and the benefits of being part of a supportive group are an added bonus.
- It is important for those of us in need of help to own up to our difficulties, but not to rely totally on another person, or work group to resolve them.

Under the UK Health and Safety at Work Act, each of us in the workplace has a duty of care to ensure that we do not put ourself or our colleagues or staff at risk, or cause them harm by our behaviour or actions. In essence, building and developing a supportive culture at work is simply an extension of this duty of care.

Exercise and stress control

Taking regular physical exercise, to expend the pent-up energy produced by the stress response is effective and one of the most used methods of stress management. An exercise routine should not be exhausting, punishing or aggressive. Regular activities such as walking, dancing, cycling and swimming can contribute to a fitness programme and help to control stress. It must be remembered that exercise is also a stressor, and that tough, competitive exercise can increase stress levels and be dangerous when not monitored by professional trainers and advisors.

Type A coronary-prone doctors should also keep in mind that they are usually very good at starting an exercise programme because of their goal-driven style of behaviour. Sadly, work tends to dominate their lives and so the well-intentioned plan to join AND USE a health club or fitness centre is likely to fail. This situation creates an additional source of stress because it becomes yet another goal that the Type A individual has not realized. Problems also arise because Type As set goals for themselves that are unrealistic. Typically, they announce their intention to join a health club and visit it every day, either before or after work! At the end of a 3-week period they realize that they have attended the gym only on two occasions because work has come first. Since they usually go to work earlier and stay later than everyone else, the likelihood of taking exercise before or after work was always a remote and unachievable goal. Nevertheless, research evidence gives credence to the idea that exercise is good for the body and the mind.

Our increasingly sedentary lifestyle, both at work and at home, is acknowledged as a contributory factor to ill health.

- Heart disease occurs almost twice as often in the inactive person compared to the highly active. Physical inactivity is an acknowledged risk factor for coronary heart disease (CHD) (Griffiths 1996)
- A sedentary lifestyle increases the risk of CHD to a similar extent as established risk factors of hypertension, high serum cholesterol and cigarette smoking (Berlin & Colditz 1990). Many studies have demonstrated the links between physical activity, blood pressure and cholesterol levels, and physical activity is an important protective factor in CHD (Shaper & Wannamethee 1991).
- Research also provides increasing evidence for the premise that exercise is associated with a reduced incidence of other physical problems (Ashton 1993). For example, more than 15 epidemiological studies suggested an increased risk of colon cancer among the physically inactive. In men, high levels of physical activity may provide some protection against prostate cancer, while in

women, exercise may protect against cancer of the breast and of the cervix, uterus and ovaries. Exercise also plays a role in minimizing the impact and in the management of osteoporosis, inflammatory joint diseases, such as rheumatoid arthritis and ankylosing spondylitis, and lower back pain.

- Exercise also improves our quality of sleep and may increase an individual's tolerance to the need to work unsocial hours and shift work (Ashton 1993, Härmä 1996). The majority of regular exercisers also report less depression, stress, fatigue and aggression (Ashton 1993), although much research has failed unequivocally to support the hypothesis that exercise is a causal factor in good psychological health. Thus, it is important to note that there is a difference between physical fitness and physical activity, and it seems likely that physical activity has a positive effect on psychological health and mood (Thirlaway & Benton 1996)

- Exercise may be beneficial, both physiologically and psychologically, in the prevention and rehabilitation of alcohol abuse (Svebak 1996).

It appears that moderate physical exercise reduces physical reactivity to stress, and it is also possible that fit individuals may be less psychologically reactive in stressful situations. Whilst some studies have shown that attendance on an exercise fitness programme can reduce levels of anxiety and depression and improve mood states, the benefits of the increased social interactions that can result from regular exercise activities with other people cannot be ignored. Thus, exercise is viewed as a coping mechanism that reduces the physiological consequences of exposure to stress. Therefore:

1. Engaging in long-term aerobic exercise may decrease the level of physiological arousal that occurs during stressful situations.
2. Exercise during a stressful event will discharge the physical excitation build-up; that is the metabolism of fatty acids released into the bloodstream, etc.

3. Exercise activity may induce a state of relaxation and help to improve one's self-esteem.
4. Incorporating regular physical activity into a work schedule will help you to relax, feel better, be more mellow and have more energy (Cejka 1999).
5. Moderate aerobic exercise is associated with improvements in perceived ability to cope with stress and with reductions in tension, anxiety and depression (Steptoe et al. 1988). The psychological improvement may emerge from factors such as the sense of achievement, mastery and personal self-control.

Aerobic exercise has received much praise as a stress antidote, however, brisk walking, jogging, energetic dancing and swimming are a few alternatives suggested as part of a stress-management programme. Even comparatively moderate forms of exercise, such as brisk walking, are associated with a lower level of morbidity and mortality due to CHD. Whilst exercise should not be exhausting or aggressive, sports such as squash and tennis are excellent ways of releasing tension and frustration (see the section above on venting steam). Further, it is suggested that the Type A individual should try to take part in exercise activity which involves other people in order to maximize the opportunity to build and develop the social support networks that are often neglected. However, Type As must refrain from introducing an aggressive or highly competitive element into group or team activities because it will further exacerbate their 'need to win' behaviour, and create frustrations if they lose!

There are some risks associated with exercise, namely sudden cardiac death, musculoskeletal injuries, disturbances of temperature regulation (Ashton 1993), immunodepression and exercise addiction or dependency (Griffiths 1996). Also, intensive exercise training has been shown to reduce a range of immune parameters that protect against infection and thereby increase susceptibility to illness (for example, secretory immunoglobin-A, Bristow, cited in Wetherall 2002). Therefore, any advice to take more exercise must always include a check-up on one's fitness levels before embarking on new, unfamiliar or strenuous activity. Professional advice is invaluable in avoiding sports and exercise injuries. Nevertheless, we must acknowledge that just the thought of this type of physical activity would be a major source of stress to certain individuals. Fortunately, physical activity in the form of gardening, a game of golf, cleaning the car or doing vigorous housework can also reduce the negative impact of a sedentary work life. It will also remove the workaholic doctor or Type A doctor from the medical practice work environment, into leisure, social and family activities.

Career breaks

The opportunity to take a career sabbatical can help a doctor to recover from the effects of exposure to stress, preferably before becoming a 'victim' of stress and burnout. With so many doctors working to the point of exhaustion, more medical professionals should be encouraged to take career breaks and sabbaticals. Ideally, this strategy should be used before the individual becomes a casualty of exposure to stress because the prevention of stress-related problems is desirable, more likely to be effective and more cost-effective than waiting until a need exists to cure a casualty of mismanaged stress. However, a career break can also be used to help the doctor to reflect on their next career steps if they have come to a professional crossroads. Whilst a short sabbatical of 1 or 2 months can be beneficial, some individuals need up to 1 year to fully recharge themselves. Sabbaticals should not be tied to grade or length of service, but should reflect the need of the medical professional to help them adapt and cope with a rapidly changing and demanding healthcare environment. Given the high cost of replacing talent and experience, this can be a highly effective strategy for retaining doctors who may otherwise leave the profession.

Conclusion

We believe that it is important to avoid the preoccupation with stress as a negative concept. NOT ALL STRESS IS BAD – but mismanaged stress is damaging in its consequences! If the healthcare system and doctors persist in blaming stress for all ills and using stress as a whipping boy, it is likely that we will continue to deny stress and react to the management of stress-inducing problems in an ineffective and negative manner. In such circumstances the symptoms of stress are often ignored until a harmful condition arises and the doctor becomes a casualty of mismanaged stress.

The person who chooses to become a medical practitioner is seeking a challenging, demanding and satisfying job. Stress has been described as 'challenge, variety and the spice of life'; it is unwanted stress that is damaging and harmful – and the kiss of death! The profession of doctor and medical practice offer challenge and stimulation and a great deal of satisfaction from a job done well. Mastery of difficult situations, variety, and coping with the responsibility for the good health and life of another person are all positive features of the job that can provide tremendous job satisfaction. It is likely that this protects the doctor from some of the negative and stressful aspects of the job. Indeed, any successful stress-management programme must emphasize the positives and build on these aspects of the job or a satisfying home and personal life. It is important to stay focussed on the best things about medical practice, as well the worst things about being a doctor, when attempting to diagnose and identify stress. Ultimately, the management of stress requires us to balance the good with the bad.

In the UK, the NHS is the largest employer in Britain, and healthcare workers and doctors are susceptible to stress because of the nature of their work. As we have observed, surveys suggest that stress is endemic within the NHS (Rees & Cooper 1992), and there is evidence to suggest that this problem persists across Continental Europe, North America, Canada and Japan (Smith 2000). In addition to the strains and pressures of caring for more and more patients, diminished professional status, loss of autonomy, and wider strategic and societal change have added to the stress burden of medical practitioners. Patients have become consumers and doctors have become service providers. The future continues to look uncertain and characterized by change – and change, whether positive or negative, is potentially stressful. In fact, as we write, a consultant surgeon is being interviewed on the radio – he is complaining because he currently must answer to twenty-two separate bodies in the process of monitoring, data gathering, inspection, and appraisal – and some sets of forms can take between 15 and 20 hours to complete! Also, the NHS appraisal process requires him to be interviewed by his peers and to take part in the interview process of peers; in addition he must submit lengthy documentation in order to be re-validated by the General Medical Council. All of this takes time away from seeing patients and detracts from his goal of the delivery of a good healthcare service. He says that every time there is an incident, another regulatory body seems to appear – there is no trust – and he and his colleagues are completely demoralized. It is very apparent that medical practitioners must take personal action to minimize the strains and pressures that are an inevitable part of work in medical practice. Whilst mismanaged stress can be harmful and can lead to burnout, much can be done to prevent it.

In the past, doctors were expected to plan their professional and domestic lives in line with William Osler's view of a medical career:

Heavy as are your responsibilities to those nearest and dearest, they are outweighed by the responsibilities to yourself, to the profession and to the public, (Osler 1903).

This philosophy and the subsequent direction of medical practice have become too costly to doctors, their families, patients and the healthcare system itself. Over a century since Osler outlined these principles for the practice of medicine, initiatives are finally being directed at increasing the size of the medical workforce and promoting family-friendly policies and retainer schemes (White 1998, Department of Health 1999, Dumelow 2000). In addition, counselling schemes and employee assistance programmes are in place for doctors, medical practice staff and patients. Many authorities and organizations offer stress-management courses for doctors, and the World Wide Web is used to provide valuable information on stress management (for example the Texas Medical Association – cited in Murray 2000). Drug and alcohol policies are also implemented in a number of medical schools (Williams 1999). However, there is still an urgent need for doctors to adopt a self-management approach to stress because this is still 'all too little' and not comprehensive enough to avoid the complex stress-related problems reported by medical practitioners. As Kirkcaldy et al. (2000) have shown, there is a need for awareness of personal stressors as well as specific medical workload stressors. Medical settings are not uniform, professionally or occupationally and within each speciality the individual doctor can display different ways of perceiving and construing a potential stressor situation. Stress prevention should be aimed primarily at balancing job- and home-life demands. But, successful stress control requires a systematic approach and the 'Triple A' stress-management model provided guides this process. Remember, in this instance, 'Triple A' is not the 'American Alcoholics Association', but the management of stress through the processes of AWARENESS, ANALYSIS and ACTION.

Understanding why we need to change certain aspects of our behaviour and work environment is the first step in a stress-management programme, knowing what to change is the next. We hope that you will be able to take time to apply some of the guidelines, tips and options described in this book to self-manage stress, and optimize your effectiveness, satisfaction and happiness as a medical practitioner and carer of others.

References

Adair JA 1982 Effective time management. Pan, London

Albrecht K 1979 Stress and the manager: making it work for you. Prentice Hall, New Jersey

Allen J, Bor R 1997 Counselling. In: Baum A, Newman S, Weinman J, West R, McManus C (eds) Cambridge handbook of psychology, health and medicine Cambridge University Press, Cambridge, pp. 206–209

Allibone A, Oakes D, Shannon HS 1981 The health and health care of doctors. Journal of the Royal College of General Practitioners 31: 728–734

Arnetz BB, Akerstedt T, Anderzen I 1990 Sleepiness in physicians on night call duty. Work and Stress 4: 71–73

Ashton D 1993 Exercise: health benefits and risks. European Occupational Health Series No. 7. World Health Organization, Copenhagen

Bailey R, Clarke M 1989 Stress and coping in nursing. Chapman and Hall, London

Baldwin PJ, Newton RW, Buckley G, Roberts MA, Dodd M 1997 Senior house officers in medicine: postal survey of training and work experience. British Medical Journal 314: 740–743

Beck AT, Emery G, Greenberg RI 1985 Anxiety disorders and phobias. Basic Books, New York

Beck AT 1987 Cognitive models of depression. Journal of Cognitive Psychotherapy 1: 5–37

Beckman H, Markakis K, Suchman S, Frankel R 1994 The doctor-patient relationship and malpractice. Archives of International Medicine 154: 1365–1370

Beecham L 2000 BMA warns of stress suffered by senior doctors. British Medical Journal (Medicopolitical Digest) July 1

Beehr TA, Newman JE 1978 Job stress, employee health and organizational effectiveness: A facet analysis model and literature review. Personnel Psychology 31: 665–699

Berlin JA, Colditz GA 1990 A meta-analysis of physical activity in the prevention of coronary heart disease. American Journal of Epidemiology 132: 612–628

Bortner RW 1969 A short rating scale as a potential measure of pattern A behaviour. Journal of Chronic Diseases 22: 87–91

Bower P, West R, Tylee A, Hann M 1999 Patients' perceptions of the role of the general practitioner in the management of emotional problems. British Journal of Health Psychology 4: 41–52

Branton P, Oborne DJ 1979 A behavioural study of anaesthetists at work. In: Oborne DJ, Gruneberg, MM, Eiser SR (eds) Research in psychology and medicine, vol 1. Academic Press, London

British Association of Counselling 1992 Code for counsellors. British Association for Counselling, Rugby

British Medical Association 1992 Stress in the medical profession. BMA London

British Medical Association 1993 The morbidity and mortality of the medical profession. BMA, London

British Medical Journal 2000 Minerva; Nov 25

Brooke D, Edwards G, Taylor C 1991 Addiction as an occupational hazard: 144 doctors with drug and alcohol problems. British Journal of Addiction 86: 1011–1016

Bruch MH 1997 Relaxation training. In: Baum A, Newman S, Weinman J, West R, McManus C (eds) Cambridge handbook of psychology, health and medicine. Cambridge University Press, Cambridge, pp. 248–251

Burbeck R, Coomber S, Robinson SM, Todd D 2001 Occupational stress in consultants in accident and emergency medicine: a national survey of levels of stress at work. Annual Conference Proceedings: British Psychological Society August 9–2: 163

Burke RJ 2001 Job stress, work satisfaction and physician militancy. Stress and Health 17: 263–271

Burke RJ, Richardson AM 1990 Sources of satisfaction and stress among Canadian physicians. Psychological Reports 67: 1335–1344

Calnan M, Williams S 1995 Challenges to professional autonomy in the United Kingdom. Perceptions of general practitioners. International Journal of Health Services 25: 219–241

Cannon WB 1935 Stress, strain and homeostasis. American Journal of Medical Science 189-1: 1–14

Caplan RP 1994 Stress, anxiety and depression in hospital consultants, general practitioners and senior health service managers. British Medical Journal 309: 1261–1263

Carroll C, Harris MG, Ross G 1991 Haemodynamic adjustments to mental stress in normotensives and subjects with mildly elevated blood pressure. Psychophysiology 28: 438–446

Cartwright S, Anderson R 1981 General practice revisited. Tavistock, London

Carver CS, Scheier MF, Weintraub JK 1989 Assessing coping strategies: A theoretically based approach. Journal of Personality and Social Psychology 56: 267–283

Cejka S 1999 How to ban job burnout. Medical Economics Jan 11

Chambers R, Wall D, Campbell I 1996 Stresses, coping mechanisms and job satisfaction in general practitioner registrars. British Journal of General Practice 46: 343–348

Clarke IM, Morin JE, Warnell I 1994 Personality factors and the practice of anaesthesia: A psychometric evaluation. Canadian Journal of Anaesthesia 41: 393–397

Cohen S, Ashby Wills T 1985 Stress, social support and the buffering hypothesis. Pyschology Bulletin 98: 310–357

Commonwealth Fund, Harris Interactive, Harvard 2000 International health policy survey of physicians. Harvard, New York

Conroy RN, Teehan M, Siriwardena R, Smyth O, McGee HH, Fernandes P 2002 Attitudes to doctors and medicine: The effect of setting and doctor-patient relationship. British Journal of Health Psychology 7: 117–125

Cooper CL, Clarke S, Rowbottom AM 1999 Occupational stress, job satisfaction and well-being among anaesthetists. Stress Medicine 15: 115–126

Cooper CL, Cooper RD, Eaker LH 1988 Living with stress. Penguin–Health/Medicine, UK

Cooper CL, Marshall J 1978 Understanding executive stress. Macmillan, London

Cooper CL, Rout U, Faragher B 1989 Mental health, job satisfaction and job stress among general practitioners. British Medical Journal 289: 369–370

Cooper CL, Sadri G, Allison T, Reynolds P 1992 Stress counselling in the Post Office. Counselling Psychology Quarterly 3(1): 3–11

Cooper CL, Sloan SJ, Williams S 1988 Occupational stress indicator management guide. ASE, Windsor, UK

Crane M 1998 Why burned-out doctors get sued more often. Medical Economics May 26

Crown S, Crisp AH 1979 Manual of the Crown Crisp Experiential Index. Hodder & Stoughton, London

Davis H, Fallowfield L 1991 Counselling and communication in health care. John Wiley, Chichester

Department of Health 1999 Improving working lives. DoH, Wetherby

Dickson DE 1996 Editorial: Stress. Anaesthesia 51: 523–524

Deary IJ, Blenkin H, Agius RH, Endler NS, Zealley H, Wood R 1996 Models of job-related stress and personal achievement among consultant doctors. British Journal of Psychology 87: 2–3

Dobson R 2001 Stresses on women doctors may cause higher suicide risk. British Medical Journal April 21

Dumelow C 2000 Relation between a career and family life for English hospital consultants: qualitative, semi-structured interview study. British Medical Journal May 27

Edwards J, Baglioni A 1990 Stress, Type-A, coping and psychological and physical symptoms: a multi-sample test of alternative models. Human Relations 43: 919–956

Enzmann D, Schaufeli WB, Janssen P, Rozeman A 1998 Dimensionality and validity of the Burnout Measure. Journal of Occupational and Organizational Psychology 71: 331–351

Firth-Cozens J 1987 Emotional distress in junior house officers. British Medical Journal 205: 533–536

Firth Cozens J 1993 Stress, psychological problems and clinical performance. In Vincent C, Ennis M, Audley RMJ (eds) Medical accidents. Oxford University Press, Oxford

Firth-Cozens J 1998 Hours, sleep, teamwork and stress. British Medical Journal November 14

Firth-Cozens J, Morrison LA 1987 Sources of stress and ways of coping in junior house officers. Research Report SAPU No. 8873. University of Sheffield, UK

Ford CV, Wentz DK 1986 Internship: what is stressful? Southern Medical Journal 79: 595–599

Freeling P, Rao B, Paykel E, Sireling L, Burton R 1985 Unrecognised depression in general practice. British Medical Journal 290: 1880–1883

Friedman MD, Rosenman RH 1974 Type A behaviour and your heart. Knopf, New York

Galassi JP, Galassi MD, Vedder MJ 1981 Perspectives on assertion as a social skills model. In: Wine JD, Smye MD (eds) Social competence. Guildford, New York

Goldberg D, Huxley P 1992 Common mental disorders: a biosocial model. Routledge, London

Graham J, Albery IP, Ramirez AJ, Richards MA 2001 How hospital consultants cope with stress at work: implications for their mental health. Stress and Health 17: 85–89

Griffiths A 1996 The benefits of employee exercise programmes: a review. Work and Stress 10(1): 5–23

Grol R, Mokkink H, Smits A, VanEijk J, Mesker-Neisten J 1985 Work satisfaction of general practitioners and the quality of patient care. Family Practice 2: 128–135

Guppy A, Weatherstone L 1997 Coping strategies, dysfunctional attitudes and psychological well-being in white-collar public sector employees. Work and Stress 11(1); 58–67

Hannay D, Usherwood T, Platts M 1992 Workload of general practitioners before and after the new contract. British Medical Journal 304: 615–818

Härmä M 1996 Exercise, shiftwork and sleep. In: Kerr J, Griffiths A, Cox T (eds) Workplace health: employee exercise and fitness. Taylor Francis, London

Harrison R 1974 When power conflicts trigger team spirit. European Business Spring: 27–65

Heim E 1991 Job stressors and coping in health professionals. Psychotherapy and Psychosomatics 55: 90–99

Heron J 1977 Catharsis in human development. Human Potential Research Project, University of Guildford, Surrey

Howie JGR, Heaney DJ, Maxwell M, Walker JJ, Freeman GK, Rai H 1999 Quality in general practice consultations: cross sectional survey. British Medical Journal 319: 738–743

Ivancevich JM, Matteson MT 1980 Stress and work. Scott, Foresman, Illinois

Jacobson E 1929 Progressive relaxation. University of Chicago Press, Chicago

Jex SM, Bliese PD 1999 Efficacy effects as a moderator of the impact of work-related stressors: A multi-level study. Journal of Applied Psychology 84: 349–361

Jex SM, Elecqua TC 1999 Time management as a moderator of relations between stressors and strain. Work and Stress 13-2: 182–191

Kahn RL, Wolfe DM, Quinn R, Snoek JD, Rosenthal RA 1964 Organizational stress. Wiley, New York

Karasek R, Theorell T 1990 Healthy work: stress, productivity and the reconstruction of working life. Basic, New York

Kirkcaldy BD, Timpop R, Cooper CL 1997 Working hours, job stress, work satisfaction, and accident rates among medical practitioners and allied personnel. International Journal of Stress Management 4-2: 79–87

Kirkcaldy BD, Athanasou JA, Trimpop R 2000 The idiosyncratic construction of stress: examples from medical settings. Stress Medicine 16: 315–326

Kompier M, Levi L 1994 Stress at work: causes, effects and prevention. A guide for small and medium sized enterprises. European Foundation for the Improvement of Living and Working Conditions, Dublin

Kornhauser A 1965 Mental health of the industrial worker. John Wiley, New York

Lang D 1992 Preventing short-term strain through time management coping. Work and Stress 6: 169–176

Lazarus R, Folkman S 1984 Stress, appraisal and coping. Springer, New York

Leese B, Bosanquet N 1996 Changes in general practice organisation: survey of general practitioners' views on the 1990 contract and fund holding. British Journal of General Practice 46: 95–99

Leiter MP 1991 Coping patterns as predictors of burnout: The function of control and escapist coping patterns. Journal of Organizational Behaviour 12: 123–144

Leonard C, Fanning N, Attwood J, Buckley M 1998 The effect of fatigue, sleep deprivation and onerous working hours on the physical and mental well-being of pre-registration house officers. Irish Journal of Medical Science 167: 22–25

Lewis J 1997 Independent contractors. GPs and the GP contract in the post-war period. National Primary Care Research and Development Centre, Manchester

Ley P 1988 Communication with patients: improving communication, satisfaction and compliance. Chapman & Hall, London

Lichenstein RL 1998 The job satisfaction and retention of physicians in organizational settings: a literature review. Medical Care 41: 139–179

Lim VK 1997 Moderating effects of work-based support on the relationship between job security and its consequences. Work and Stress 11-3: 251–266

Lin N, Ensel WM, Simeone RS, Kuo W 1979 Social support, stressful life events and illness: A model of an empirical test. Journal of Health and Social Behaviour 20: 108–119

Macan TH 1994 Time management: test of a process model. Journal of Applied Psychology 79: 381–391

Macan TH, Shahani C, Dipboye RL, Phillips AP 1990 College students' time management: Correlations with academic performance and stress. Journal of Educational Psychology 82: 760–768

Maslach C 1993 Burnout: A multidimensional perspective. In: Schaufeli WB, Maslach C, Marek T (eds) Professional burnout: recent developments in theory and research. Taylor Francis, Washington DC, pp. 19–32

McGee HM 1998 Patient satisfaction surveys: Are they useful as indicators of quality of care? Journal of Health Gain 2: 5–8

McKee M, Black N 1993 Junior doctors' work at night: What is done and how much is appropriate? Journal of Public Health Medicine 15: 16–24

McNamee R, Kee RI, Corkhill CM 1987 Morbidity and early retirement among anaesthetists and other specialists. Anaesthesia 42: 1333–1340

Murray D 2000 How to stay sane in the crazy world of medicine. Medical Economics Jan 24

Murray RM 1976 Alcoholism among male doctors in Scotland. Lancet ii: 729–733

Myerson S 1993 The effects of policy change on family doctors: stress in general practice under the new contract. Journal of Management in Medicine 7: 7–26

Ormel J, Van Den Brink W, Koeter W, Giel R, Van Der Meek K, Van de Willige G, Wilmink F 1989 Recognition, management and outcome of psychological disorders in primary care: A naturalistic follow-up study. Psychological Medicine 20: 909–923

Osler W 1903 The principles and practice of medicine, 5th edn. Appleton-Century-Crofts, New York

Paice E, Moss F, West G, Grant J 1997 Association of use of a log book and experience as a pre-registration house officer. An interview survey. British Medical Journal 314: 213–215

Payne RL, Rick JT 1986 Psychobiological markers of stress in surgeons and anaesthetists. In: Schmidt TH, Dembroski TM, Blumchen G (eds) Biological and psychological factors in cardiovascular disease. Springer-Verlag, London

Pereira Gray D 1988 Counselling in general practice. Journal of the Royal College of General Practitioners 38: 50–51

Pines AM, Aronson E 1988 Career burnout: causes and cures. Free Press, New York

Priest R, Vize C, Roberts A, Roberts M, Tylee A 1996 Lay people's attitude to treatment of depression: Results of opinion poll for Defeat Depression campaign just before its launch. British Medical Journal 313: 858–859

Quick JC, Quick JD 1984 Organizational stress and preventive management. McGraw-Hill, New York

Ramirez AJ, Graham J, Richards MA, Cull A, Gregory WM 1996 Mental health of hospital consultants: The effects of stress and satisfaction at work. Lancet 347: 724–728

Rankin HJ, Seieys NM, Elliott-Binns CP 1987 Determinants of mood in general practitioners. British Medical Journal 295: 618–620

Read M, Draycott T, Beckwith J 1988 Night vision. Health Service Journal 5 Jan: 24–25

Rees DW 1995 Work-related stress in health service employees. Journal of Managerial Psychology 10(3): 4–11

Rees DW, Cooper CL 1992 Occupational stress in health service workers in the UK. Stress Medicine 8: 79–90

Reuben DB 1985 Depressive symptoms in medical house officers: effects of level of training and work rotation. Archives of International Medicine 145: 286–288

Richardson AM, Burke RJ 1991 Occupational stress and job satisfaction among physicians: Sex differences. Social Science and Medicine 33: 1179–1187

Richings JC, Khara GS, McDowell M 1986 Suicide in young doctors. British Journal of Psychiatry 149: 475–478

Rout U, Rout JK 1994 Job satisfaction, mental health and job stress among general practitioners before and after the new contract – a comparative study. Family Practice 11: 300–306

Rout U, Rout JK 1997 A comparative study on occupational stress, job satisfaction and mental health in British general practitioners and Canadian family physicians. Psychological Health Medicine 2: 181–190

Rout U, Rout JK 2000 Gender differences in stress, satisfaction and mental well-being among general practitioners. British Psychological Society, Annual Conference Proceedings

Royal College of General Practitioners 1996 The nature of general medical practice. Report from General Practice 27. Royal College of General Practitioners, London

Scheiber SC 1987 Stress in physicians. In: Payne R, Firth-Cozens J (eds) Stress in health care professionals. Wiley, Chichester

Schultz JH, Luthe W 1959 Autogenic training: a psychophysiological approach to psychotherapy. Grune and Stratton, New York

Scott AJ 1992 Editorial: House staff = shift workers? Journal of Occupational Medicine 34: 1161–1163

Seeley HJ 1996 The practice of anaesthesia: A stressor for the middle-aged? Anaesthesia 51: 571–574

Seyle H 1976 Stress in health and disease. Butterworth, London

Shaffer M 1983 Life after stress. Contemporary Books, Chicago

Shaper AG, Wannamethee G 1991 Physical activity and ischaemic heart disease in British middle-aged men. British Heart Journal 66: 384–394

Sibbald B, Enzer I, Cooper C, Rout U, Sutherland V 2000 GP job satisfaction I 1987, 1990, and 1998: lessons for the future? Family Practice 17-5: 364–371

Sibicky M, Dovidio JF 1986 Stigma of psychological therapy. Journal of Counselling Psychology 33: 148–154

Simpson LA, Grant L 1991 Source and magnitude of job stress among physicians. Journal of Behavioural Medicine 14-1: 27–42

Skinner BF 1969 Contingencies of reinforcement: a theoretical analysis. Appleton-Century Crofts, New York

Smith R 2000 Hamster health care: time to stop running faster and redesign health care. British Medical Journal Dec 23

Sonnetag S 1996 Work group factors and individual well-being. In: West MM (ed) Handbook of work group psychology. Wiley, Chichester

Sparks K, Cooper CL, Freid Y, Shirom A 1997 The effects of work on health: A meta-analytic review. Journal of Occupational and Organizational Psychology 70: 391–408

Sparks K, Faragher B, Cooper, CL 2001 Well-being and occupational health in the 21st century workplace.

Journal of Occupational and Organizational Psychology 74: 489–509

Spurgeon A, Harrington JM 1989 Work performance and health of junior hospital doctors: a review of the literature. Work and Stress 3: 117–128

Spurgeon A, Harrington JM, Cooper CL 1997 Health and safety problems associated with long working hours: a review of the current position. Occupational Environmental Medicine 6: 367–375

Steptoe A, Fieldman C, Evans O 1993 An experimental study of the effects of control over work pace on cardiovascular responsivity. Journal of Psychophysiology 7: 290–300

Steptoe A, Moses J, Edwards S, Mathews A 1988 Effects of aerobic conditioning on mental well-being and reactivity to stress. In: Proceedings of the Sport, Health Psychology and Exercise Symposium, Bisham Abbey National Sports Centre, Buckinghamshire. The Sports Council, London, pp. 192–201

Stevenson HM, Williams AP 1985 Physicians and Medicare: Professional ideology and Canadian health care policy. Canadian Public Policy 11: 504–521

Sutherland VJ 1995 Stress and the new contract for general practitioners. Journal of Managerial Psychology 10-3: 17–28

Sutherland VJ, Cooper CL 1992 Job stress, satisfaction and mental health among general practitioners before and after introduction of the new contract. British Medical Journal 304: 1545–1548

Sutherland VJ, Cooper CL 1993 Identifying distress among general practitioners; predictors of psychological ill-health and job dissatisfaction. Social Science and Medicine 37: 575–581

Sutherland V, Makin P, Cox C 2000 The management of safety. The behavioural approach to changing organizations. Sage, London

Svebak S 1996 Alcohol abuse, physical fitness and the prevention of relapse. In Kerr J, Griffiths A, Cox T (eds) Workplace health: employee exercise and fitness. Taylor Francis, London

Swanson V, Power K 1996 A comparison of stress and job satisfaction in female and male GPs and consultants. Stress Medicine 12: 17–26

Talbott GD, Gallegos KV, Wilson PO, Porter TL 1987 The medical association of Georgia's impaired physician programme. Review of first 1000 physicians: Analysis of speciality. Journal of American Medical Association 257-2: 227–230

Tattersall A, Bennett P, Pugh S 1999 Stress and coping in hospital doctors. Stress Medicine 15: 109–113

Thirlaway K, Benton D 1996 Exercise and mental health: the role of activity and fitness. In: Kerr J, Griffiths A, Cox T (eds) Workplace health: employee exercise and fitness. Taylor Francis, London

Torsvall L, Akerstedt T 1998 Disturbed sleep while being on-call: An EEG study of ships engineers. Sleep 11: 35–38

Touhy CJ 1976 Medical politics after Medicare: The Ontario case. Canadian Public Policy 2: 192–210

Warr P, Cook J, Wall T 1979 Scales for the measurement of some work attitudes and aspects of psychological well-being. Journal of Occupational Psychology 52: 129–148

West MA, Reynolds S 1995 Employee attitudes to work-based counselling services. Work and Stress 9(1): 31–44

Wetherall M 2002 'Not to be sneezed at.' The Psychologist 15 (6): 305

White C 1998 Mystery of "7000 extra doctors." British Medical Journal 317–300

Williams DF 1999 Drug and alcohol policies are rare at medical schools in the UK. British Medical Journal July 10

Wingfield HR, Anstey TJ 1991 Job stress in general practice: Practitioner age, sex and attitudes as predictors. Family Practice 8: 140–144

Wolf SG 1960 Cited in Lewis H, Griswold H, Underwood H,1960 (eds) Stress and heart disease: modern concepts of cardiovascular disease. American Heart Association, New York, pp. 559–603

.Appendices

Appendix I   Stress log

Stress may be perceived as a single, dramatic incident or an accumulation of less serious events. It might be interpreted as pressure, strain or tension that creates anxiety, anger, worry, guilt, or mild agitation. In fact, STRESS IS IN THE EYE OF THE BEHOLDER!
Keep this daily log in order to identify and understand stress.

1. At the end of each day, try to identify your most stressful experience. It could be a work- or home-related incident.
2. At the end of the week, complete the section about your reactions to stress and describe how you typically cope with stress.

Try to be specific about these events, the other people involved, how you felt and what happened. It also helps to try and think what you could have done differently.

Monday _____ number of hours worked

Incidents	People involved/what happened/feelings and reactions	What could have been done differently?
Work-related		
Home-related		

Tuesday _____ number of hours worked

Incidents	People involved/what happened/feelings and reactions	What could have been done differently?
Work-related		
Home-related		

Wednesday _____ number of hours worked

Incidents	People involved/what happened/feelings and reactions	What could have been done differently?
Work-related		
Home-related		

Thursday _____ number of hours worked

Incidents	People involved/what happened/feelings and reactions	What could have been been done differently?
Work-related		
Home-related		

Appendix I   *continued*

Friday _____ number of hours worked		
Incidents	People involved/what happened/feelings and reactions	What could have been done differently?
Work-related		
Home-related		

Saturday _____ number of hours worked		
Incidents	People involved/what happened/feelings and reactions	What could have been done differently?
Work-related		
Home-related		

Sunday _____ number of hours worked		
Incidents	People involved/what happened/feelings and reactions	What could have been done differently?
Work-related		
Home-related		

It does not matter on what day of the week you start the log, but at the end of a 7-day, normal work period, please complete the following questions

- How can you tell when you are feeling stressed? What feelings, reactions and behaviours do you express?
- How do you usually cope when under stress?

Appendix II   Example of a time log: Day/Date _____

Start time/duration		Activity	Time problem (Who/what/ why)	Outcome	Feelings/ reaction/ further action
0800	35 minutes	Travel to surgery			
0835	25 minutes	Surgery preparation	Surgery start late – receptionist late for work again	All appoint- ments delayed by 20 minutes – roll-over effect during day	Angry at being let down Need to resolve staff 'lateness' issue

Appendix II   *Continued*

1130	50 minutes	Deal with incoming mail	Interrupted by colleagues asking for advice	Interruption could have waited	Cross with self – should have been more assertive – less time for my lunch break
1220	40 minutes	Lunch			A shorter break than I wanted, but felt relaxed after getting away from work for a while – a good morning
1300	3 hours	Patient visits	Traffic problems – late for second appointment	Late for evening surgery!	Feel unable to schedule more time for travel – too many patients to see
1625	2 hours	Evening surgery			Surgery went well – but late finish
1900		Update patient records; plan work schedule for tomorrow	Unexpected telephone call from mother of child patient; a non-serious situation – child has appointment for next week; mother is a known worrier	Agreed to return call tomorrow at an agreed time to discuss the situation, when I have reviewed records. Mother satisfied with this plan	Felt pleased about the way I handled the unexpected call

Index

Buddy system, 134, 138, 164
Burnout, 5, 6, 58, 59–63
  costs, 61
  definition, 59
  in hospital doctors, 38
  management, 124
  prevention, 61–63
  symptoms, 59–60

C

Canada, physician militancy, 13–14,
    28–29
Cancer, physical activity and, 165–166
Career
  breaks, 124, 168
  development/achievement issues,
    21, 39
  downshift, 124
  stage, 40–41
Catecholamines, 6
Change
  dealing with, 132
  as source of stress, 13–15, 170
Chocolate consumption, 11
Chronic disease/illness, 17
Chronic stress, 103
Clutter, 74, 84–85
Co-counselling, 164
Cognitive distortion, see Faulty thinking
Cognitive reparation, 105
Cognitive restructuring, 155
Cognitive stress management methods,
    154–160
Cold extremities, 7
Collaborative behaviour, 104
Competitive behaviour, 119
Complaints, patient, 43, 45
Compromise, 104
Computerized diaries/organizers/
    planners, 86
Computers, 86–89
Conditioning, 92–93
Confidentiality, counselling services,
    140
Conflict
  benefits, 103, 104

  understanding, 102–104
Consultants, hospital
  coping strategies, 12–13
  social support by, 161
  stress in, 38–39, 170
  time pressures, 57
Consumerism, 44–45
Control (autonomy)
  GPs, 42, 43
  hospital doctors, 39, 40
  importance of, 142–143
  Type A behaviour and, 119
  work environment, 78, 80–81, 83
Coping styles/strategies
  adaptive, 10, 135–136
  cognitive, 154–158
  developing flexible, 132–133
  maladaptive, 10–13, 17, 135–136
  role of exercise, 166–167
  understanding own, 134–136
Coronary heart disease (CHD), 165
Cortisol, 6, 7
Couch potato syndrome, 11
Counselling services, 162, 171
  for GPs, 36
  using, 138–142
  see also Employee assistance
    programmes
Critical-incident analysis, 23, 24–25
Criticism, 108–111
  giving, 110–111
  receiving, 109–110
Crown Crisp Experiential Index (CCEI),
    28

D

Delegation, 74, 130
Demand, perceived versus actual, 16–17
Denial, 12, 102, 160
  stress/burnout, 60
Depression, 37
  in GPs, 23, 34
  in hospital doctors, 41
Diagnosis of stress, 1, 19–51
  process, 23–29
  techniques and methods, 23–24